Modern Concepts in Aesthetic Dentistry and Multi-disciplined Reconstructive Grand Rounds

Editors

JOHN R. CALAMIA
RICHARD D. TRUSHKOWSKY
STEVEN B. DAVID
MARK S. WOLFF

DENTAL CLINICS OF NORTH AMERICA

www.dental.theclinics.com

July 2015 • Volume 59 • Number 3

ELSEVIER

1600 John F. Kennedy Boulevard ● Suite 1800 ● Philadelphia, Pennsylvania, 19103-2899

http://www.dental.theclinics.com

DENTAL CLINICS OF NORTH AMERICA Volume 59, Number 3
July 2015 ISSN 0011-8532, ISBN: 978-0-323-39094-1

Editor: John Vassallo; j.vassallo@elsevier.com
Developmental Editor: Barbara Cohen-Kligerman

Dental Clinics of North America (ISSN 0011-8532) is published quarterly by Elsevier Inc., 360 Park Avenue South, New York, NY 10010-1710. Months of issue are January, April, July, and October. Business and Editorial Offices: 1600 John F. Kennedy Boulevard, Suite 1800, Philadelphia, PA 19103-2899. Periodicals postage paid at New York, NY and additional mailing offices. Subscription prices are $280.00 per year (domestic individuals), $485.00 per year (domestic institutions), $135.00 per year (domestic students/residents), $340.00 per year (Canadian individuals), $628.00 per year (Canadian institutions), $410.00 per year (international individuals), $628.00 per year (international institutions), and $200.00 per year (international and Canadian students/residents). International air speed delivery is included in all *Clinics* subscription prices. All prices are subject to change without notice. **POSTMASTER:** Send address changes to *Dental Clinics of North America*, Elsevier Health Sciences Division, Subscription Customer Service, 3251 Riverport Lane, Maryland Heights, MO 63043. **Customer Service (orders, claims, online, change of address): Elsevier Health Sciences Division, Subscription Customer Service, 3251 Riverport Lane, Maryland Heights, MO 63043. Tel: 1-800-654-2452 (U.S. and Canada). Fax: 314-447-8029. E-mail: journalscustomerservice-usa@elsevier.com (for print support); journalsonlinesupport-usa@elsevier.com (for online support).**

Reprints. For copies of 100 or more, of articles in this publication, please contact the Commercial Reprints Department, Elsevier Inc., 360 Park Avenue South, New York, NY 10010-1710. Tel.: 212-633-3874; Fax: 212-633-3820; E-mail: reprints@elsevier.com.

The *Dental Clinics of North America* is covered in *MEDLINE/PubMed (Index Medicus), Current Contents/Clinical Medicine, ISI/BIOMED* and *Clinahl*.

Printed in the United States of America.

Contributors

EDITORS

JOHN R. CALAMIA, DMD, FAGD
Director of the Aesthetics Honors Program, Full Professor, and Director of Aesthetic Dentistry for the Department of Cariology and Comprehensive Care, New York University College of Dentistry, New York, New York; Former Board of Director, American Academy of Cosmetic Dentistry, Madison, Wisconsin

RICHARD D. TRUSHKOWSKY, DDS
Clinical Professor; Associate Director, Advanced Program for International Dentists in Aesthetic Dentistry, Department of Cariology and Comprehensive Care, New York University College of Dentistry, New York, New York

STEVEN B. DAVID, DMD
Director, Advanced Program for International Dentists in Aesthetic Dentistry; Clinical Professor, Department of Cariology and Comprehensive Care, NYU College of Dentistry, New York, New York

MARK S. WOLFF, DDS, PhD
Professor and Chair, Associate Dean, Department of Cariology and Comprehensive Care, New York University College of Dentistry, New York, New York

AUTHORS

JAAFAR ALI, DDS
Honor's Aesthetics Student, New York University College of Dentistry, New York, New York

ZAINAB ALSADAH, BDS
Postgraduate Education Student, Advanced Program for International Dentists in Aesthetic Dentistry, New York University College of Dentistry, New York, New York

MICHAEL APA, DDS
Partner, Rosenthal Apa Group; Clinical Assistant Professor, Department of Cariology and Comprehensive Care, New York University College of Dentistry, New York, New York

DAVID MONTALVO ARIAS, DDS
Fellow, Advanced Program for International Dentists in Aesthetic Dentistry, New York University College of Dentistry, New York, New York

SAMEERA BABAR, DDS
General dentist, Peninsula Dental Center Salisbury, Maryland

LUIS M. BREA, DDS
Faculty, Advanced Program for International Dentists in Aesthetic Dentistry; Clinical Assistant Professor, Department of Cariology and Comprehensive Care, New York University College of Dentistry, New York, New York

CHRISTINE CALAMIA, DDS
Instructor, CDE Implant Program, New York University School of Dentistry, New York, New York

JOHN R. CALAMIA, DMD, FAGD
Director of the Aesthetics Honors Program, Full Professor, and Director of Aesthetic Dentistry for the Department of Cariology and Comprehensive Care, New York University College of Dentistry, New York, New York; Former Board of Directors, American Academy of Cosmetic Dentistry, Madison, Wisconsin

VINCENT CALAMIA, DDS
Private Practice, New York, New York

BRIAN CHADROFF, DDS
Private Practice; Clinical Associate Professor, Department of Periodontics and Implant Dentistry, New York University College of Dentistry, New York, New York

STEVEN B. DAVID, DMD
Director, Advanced Program for International Dentists in Aesthetic Dentistry; Clinical Professor, Department of Cariology and Comprehensive Care, New York University College of Dentistry, New York, New York

NICHOLAS J. GIANNUZZI, DDS
Case Mentor; Assistant Clinical Professor, NYU Honors Program in Aesthetics, Department of Cariology and Comprehensive Care, New York University College of Dentistry, New York City, New York

CHIANN FAN GIBSON, DMD, AAACD
Adjunct Research Instructor, Department of Prosthodontics, Tufts School of Dental Medicine, Boston, Massachusetts; Private Practice, Restorative Dentistry, Naperville, Illinois

KATERYNA GRYTSENKO, DDS
Resident, New York University College of Dentistry, New York, New York

ZAHID JUMA, DDS
Fellow, International Dental Implant Association; Coast Dental, Deland, Florida

DEAN E. KOIS, DMD, MSD
Kois Center, LLC, Seattle, Washington

JOHN C. KOIS, DMD, MSD
Professor, Graduate Prosthodontics Department, University of Washington; Kois Center, LLC, Seattle, Washington

DIANA KUKLERIS, DDS
Private Practice, Schertz, Texas

ARNOLD I. LIEBMAN, DDS
Faculty in Esthetics Honors, Department of Cariology and Comprehensive Care, New York University College of Dentistry, New York, New York

KENNETH S. MAGID, DDS, FICD
Associate Clinical Professor, International Esthetic and High Technology; Assistant Director Honors Esthetics; Director Pre-doctoral Laser Dentistry, Department of Cariology and Comprehensive Care, New York University College of Dentistry, New York, New York

SABRINA MAGID-KATZ, DMD
Clinical Instructor, Department of Cariology and Comprehensive Care, New York University College of Dentistry, New York, New York

GEORGE A. MANDELARIS, DDS, MS
Private Practice, Periodontal Medicine and Surgical Specialists, Ltd, Oakbrook Terrace, Illinois; Adjunct Clinical Assistant Professor, Department of Graduate Periodontics, University of Illinois College of Dentistry, Chicago, Illinois

THEO MANTZIKOS, DDS
Private Practice, White Plains, New York

ANDI-JEAN MIRO, DDS
Clinical Instructor, Department of Cariology and Comprehensive Care, New York University College of Dentistry, New York, New York

RAMIRO MORALES, DMD
Orthodontist, Orthodontics Program, New York University College of Dentistry, New York, New York

SHAWN DAVAIE MOTLAGH, DDS
Private Practice, Irvine, California

ANABELLA OQUENDO, DDS
Faculty, Advanced Program for International Dentists in Aesthetic Dentistry, Clinical Assistant Professor, Department of Cariology and Comprehensive Care, New York University College of Dentistry, New York, New York

ALEXANDRIA PANTZIS, DDS
Private Practice, New York, New York

MANILA NUCHHE PRADHAN, DDS
General Dentist, Private Practice, Houston, Texas

ALEX SHALMAN, DDS
Clinical Instructor, Department of Cariology and Comprehensive Care, New York University College of Dentistry, New York, New York

BARBARA SLASKA, DDS
Faculty in Esthetics Honors, Department of Cariology and Comprehensive Care, New York University College of Dentistry, New York, New York

JERRY M. SORREL, DMD
Clinical Professor, Department of Orthodontics, New York University College of Dentistry

RICHARD D. TRUSHKOWSKY, DDS
Associate Clinical Professor; Associate Director, Advanced Program for International Dentists in Esthetic Dentistry, Department of Cariology and Comprehensive Care, New York University College of Dentistry, New York, New York

DANIEL H. WARD, DDS, FAGD, FACD, FICD
Former Assistant Clinical Professor, Section of Restorative and Prosthetic Dentistry, The Ohio State University, College of Dentistry; Private Practice Columbus, Ohio

MARK S. WOLFF, DDS, PhD
Professor and Chair, Associate Dean, Department of Cariology and Comprehensive Care, New York University College of Dentistry, New York, New York

Contents

> This article updates a simple checklist of foundational knowledge in
> aesthetic dental concepts that allows clinicians to organize their thoughts,
> to record the concerns of the patient, and to map out those improvements
> that must be addressed. This adjunct is called a Smile Evaluation Form.
> Along with other adjuncts such as radiographs, study casts, and diag-
> nostic wax-ups, the Smile Evaluation Form allows clinicians to form a
> conceptual visualization of the expected end point. It provides a checklist
> for discussions with other disciplines in the team, to provide a logical
> sequence of treatment with a mutually agreed-on end point.

> This article describes a multidisciplinary approach to a functional and
> aesthetic rehabilitation. In this case study, we successfully corrected an
> anterior open bite and an exaggerated curve of Spee using restorative mo-
> dalities while still maintaining a highly aesthetic outcome. The maxillary
> anterior teeth no longer appear to have a disproportional width/length ratio
> and are now in harmony with the mandibular veneers. Posterior function
> was re-established, mostly with implant-retained crowns. Occlusal har-
> mony and stability are maintained through cuspid guidance and anterior
> disclusion. Proper selection of final restorative materials is imperative for
> the long-term survival of the restorations.

> This case report points out the previous restorative breakdown of tooth #8.
> An interdisciplinary approach had to be applied to prepare the final treat-
> ment plan. All factors were taken into account when choosing the type of
> restorations and materials in this case. The ultimate treatment is presented
> with the final result. The objectives were to clinically assess patient's cur-
> rent chief complaint, address her aesthetic needs, apply an interdisci-
> plinary approach, deliver treatment of utmost quality, and maintain oral
> health.

Proportional smile design is a useful tool for evaluating and designing smiles that are in harmony with the face. Although not always observed in nature, the recurring esthetic dental proportion is preferred by dentists surveyed to the width proportions observed in nature with normal-length teeth. The width/length ratio of the central incisor is a key determinant in providing a smile that is pleasing to dentists. Using the desired tooth length while maintaining the preferred 78% width/length ratio of the central incisor in conjunction with the recommended recurring esthetic dental proportion is a good method for designing a smile balanced with the face.

A cosmetic smile makeover has become a sought after procedure in our esthetically driven society. To promote patient satisfaction with treatment outcomes, all parties involved, including the patient, must be aware of the results that can be achieved and what is required to achieve them. Although treatment can be redone, it cannot be undone. Therefore, much patient input must be solicited and considered before beginning treatment and before the final restorations are cemented. This article provides a treatment sequence that minimizes the possibility of an unhappy patient.

Missing teeth in the esthetic zone, whether congenital or as a result of other factors, present difficult choices in clinical management. The missing teeth can be replaced by surgical or restorative intervention but are often treated orthodontically. These repositioned teeth often lead to an unaesthetic result because of differences in morphology, color, and particularly in gingival architecture. This article describes the use of multiple lasers for periodontal modification and feldspathic porcelain veneers to achieve a highly esthetic result.

This article demonstrates the use of a smile evaluation form as an adjunct in arriving at diagnosis and developing a treatment plan for a patient desiring diastema closure. It also shows the importance of the diagnostic wax-up for temporization and visualization of case outcome. The case also demonstrates the use of soft tissue lasers to create a gingival harmony that enhances the resulting esthetics. Feldspathic porcelain was used for the final restorations because they provide optimal esthetics and translucency.

This case report presents an interdisciplinary approach to achieve functioning occlusion and an aesthetically pleasing smile. This patient's concerns were spacing between upper front teeth and a gummy smile. The case was evaluated, and treatment was planned using a multidisciplinary approach. The patient rejected the option of orthognathic surgery to correct a skeletal problem. Treatment included orthodontics, osteoplasty, gingivoplasty, and porcelain veneer restorations to achieve the desired aesthetic result. Comprehensive orthodontics resulted in a functionally stable occlusion. Space distribution between maxillary anterior teeth with adequate overjet and overbite relationships allowed for conservative preparation to receive porcelain veneer restorations.

The standards of dentistry are being elevated, with a greater emphasis being placed on esthetics along with functionality. Minimally invasive dentistry has become an essential component in creating restorations that are functional and have increased longevity. In the case discussed in this article, the patient underwent 9 months of orthodontic therapy to correct her improper overbite and overjet, and the spacing of her dentition so the teeth could be positioned for future minimally invasive restorations. Orthodontic therapy was paramount in positioning the teeth so that the future restorations would have ideal axial inclinations and be as minimally invasive as possible.

Previously dentists focused on repair and maintenance of function. However, the emphasis of many patients and dentists is now on aesthetics. Often there is a need for the disciplines of orthodontics, periodontics, restorative dentistry, and maxillofacial surgery to work together in order to achieve optimum results. Currently the sequencing planning process begins with aesthetics and then function, structure, and ultimately biology.

Gummy smile cases are always esthetically demanding cases. This article presents a patient treated with an interdisciplinary treatment approach and Digital Smile Approach (DSA) using Keynote (DSA), to predictably achieve an esthetic outcome for a patient with gummy smile. The importance of using questionnaires and checklists to facilitate the gathering of diagnostic data cannot be overemphasized. The acquired data must then be transferred to the design of the final restorations. The use of digital smile design has emerged as a powerful tool in cosmetic dentistry to help both practitioner and patient visualize the final outcome.

Preface

Modern Concepts in Aesthetic Dentistry and Multidisciplined Reconstructive Grand Rounds

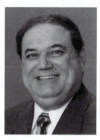 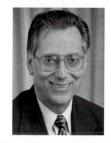 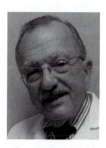 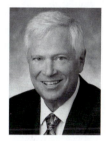

| John R. Calamia, DMD | Richard D. Trushkowsky, DDS | Steven B. David, DMD | Mark S. Wolff, DDS, PhD |

Editors

In April 2007, Elsevier published an issue of *Dental Clinics of North America* entitled "Successful Esthetic and Cosmetic Dentistry for the Modern Dental Practice." Authors and topics were selected that would provide generalists, specialists, seasoned practitioners, and recent graduates with foundational knowledge in a clear and concise text to help them provide their patients with those often elective procedures requested in the modern-day practice of dentistry.

In April 2011, with our next project, entitled "Esthetic and Cosmetic Dentistry for Modern Dental Practice: Update 2011," we continued to provide the readership with updated information on additional foundational material not covered in the previous issue. We also provided adjuncts for patient evaluation and improved communicative skills that would allow for better diagnosis, better treatment planning, better case presentation, and better laboratory communication.

In this, our third project for *Dental Clinics of North America*, entitled "Modern Concepts in Aesthetic Dentistry and Multidisciplined Reconstructive Grand Rounds," we have again provided foundational knowledge on adjuncts that will help clinicians provide quality, long-lasting restorations for their patients. In addition to this continued evidence-based information—including an updated Smile Evaluation Form, the use of the Kois analyzer, and Dr Ward's proportional smile design—this issue champions "the medical model," presenting numerous cases that apply all of our previous preparation with the intent of bringing our readers' clinical knowledge to new heights. These cases furnish not only the functional and physiologic requirements of treatment planning but also the aesthetic component that is often considered a key component of excellence in modern dental care. They each offer pearls of information that in our opinion can be immediately incorporated into the practices of readers.

Dent Clin N Am 59 (2015) xiii–xiv
http://dx.doi.org/10.1016/j.cden.2015.04.003
0011-8532/15/$ – see front matter © 2015 Published by Elsevier Inc.

dental.theclinics.com

I would like to express my sincere thanks to those rising stars as well as the nationally and internationally respected, dedicated professionals among our authors who have, without financial reward, given their time and shared their expertise in providing members of their profession with up-to-date information to assure the best clinical results are realized by dentists, technicians, and, of most importance, their patients.

I would also like to thank my coeditors, Dr Mark Wolff, Dr Richard Truskowsky, and new team member, Dr Steven David, for their help in editing as well as their written contributions to this text. Finally, I want to thank my family: my parents, Vincent J. Calamia and Sina Calamia, my wife, Sonia Calamia, DDS, my daughter, Christine Calamia-Levitsky, DDS, my son-in-law, William Levitsky, my son, Vincent Calamia, DDS, and his soon-to-be wife, Eileen Dano, DDS, for putting up with me when I take on a project as important as this issue, since it always means less time I can spend with my loved ones.

John R. Calamia, DMD
Department of Cariology and Comprehensive Care
New York University College of Dentistry
New York, NY 10010, USA

American Academy of Cosmetic Dentistry
402 West Wilson Street
Madison, WI 53703, USA

Richard D. Trushkowsky, DDS
NYU College of Dentistry
Department of Cariology and Comprehensive Care
345 East 24th Street
New York, NY 10010, USA

Steven B. David, DMD
NYU College of Dentistry
Department of Cariology and Comprehensive Care
345 East 24th Street
New York, NY 10010, USA

Mark S. Wolff, DDS, PhD
NYU College of Dentistry
Department of Cariology and Comprehensive Care
345 East 24th Street
New York, NY 10010, USA

E-mail addresses:
jrc1@nyu.edu (J.R. Calamia)
rt587@nyu.edu (R.D. Trushkowsky)
sbd3@nyu.edu (S.B. David)
mark.wolff@nyu.edu (M.S. Wolff)

The Components of Smile Design

New York University Smile Evaluation Form Revisited, Update 2015

John R. Calamia, DMD[a,b,*], Mark S. Wolff, DDS, PhD[a]

KEYWORDS

- Smile design • Treatment planning • Evaluation form

KEY POINTS

- The Smile Evaluation Form is a simple checklist of foundational knowledge in aesthetic dental concepts that allows clinicians to organize their thoughts, to record in an orderly fashion the concerns of the patient and the patient's existing problems, and to practically map out those improvements that must be addressed.

- On the completion of the Smile Evaluation Form, the clinician generally has a starting point in understanding the patient's problems, and also an end point of what is needed to be changed in order to provide a predictable aesthetic result for that patient.

- Along with other adjuncts, such as radiographs, study casts, and diagnostic wax-ups, the Smile Evaluation Form allows clinicians to form a conceptual visualization of the expected end point.

- The Smile Evaluation Form provides a checklist to refer to in discussions with other disciplines in the team, to provide a logical sequence of treatment with a mutually agreed-on end point.

INTRODUCTION

In the modern practice of dentistry, it is no longer acceptable to just repair individual teeth. More and more patients are demanding a final appearance that is not only physiologically and mechanically sound but also esthetically pleasing.[1] In addition to restoring and reconstructing the broken-down dentition, bleaching, bonding, and veneering have created possibilities for a wide variety of elective dental treatments for the purposes of enhancing appearance and often reversing the visual signs of aging.[2,3] The initial consultation visit is extremely important in understanding the chief

Disclosure: The authors have nothing to disclose.
[a] Department of Cariology and Comprehensive Care, New York University College of Dentistry, New York, NY 10010, USA; [b] Board of Directors American Academy of Cosmetic Dentistry
* Corresponding author. 1 Amherst Place, Massapequa, NY 11758.
E-mail address: jrc1@nyu.edu

Dent Clin N Am 59 (2015) 529–546
http://dx.doi.org/10.1016/j.cden.2015.03.013
0011-8532/15/$ – see front matter © 2015 Elsevier Inc. All rights reserved.

dental.theclinics.com

concerns of the patient and recording as much information as possible to allow the doctor to decide whether it is possible to provide what the patient is looking for. The author has found that, with the help of the Smile Evaluation Form,[4,5] the doctor can formulate the patient's basic problems and can quickly describe to the patient those discrepancies from the norm. The patient has a sense of what needs to be done and the doctor can explain what other adjuncts are needed to complete the best course of treatment. This form has gone a long way to communicating patients' needs, and patients can more easily decide on accepting the need for radiographs, study casts, and possible diagnostic wax-ups of the expected result.

The first part of the form (**Fig. 1**A) allows patients to indicate whether they are interested in any change to their existing smile. If the answer to this question is yes, then it

A

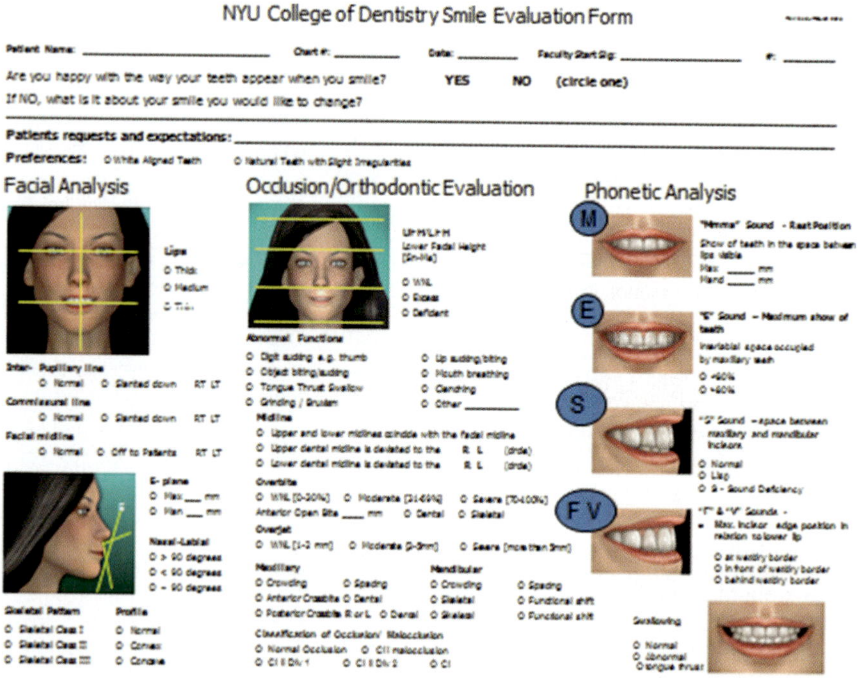

B

1. Are you happy with the way your teeth appear when you smile?   YES   NO   (circle one)

2. If NO, what is it about your smile you would like to change?_____

3. Patient's requests and expectations: _____
    Please check your preferences:

        White aligned teeth
        Natural teeth with slight irregularities

Fig. 1. (*A*) Smile Evaluation Form (side A). Updated January 2015. (*B*) Three important questions at the top of the Smile Evaluation Form. For question 2, the patient is generally given a mirror and a plastic instrument, and asked to point to areas of concern.

is left to the patient to describe what their chief concerns might be. Patients may not be able to identify their needs in other than short sentences. It is at this juncture that clinicians must decide whether the expectations of the patient are reasonable and whether the possible treatment needed is within their area of expertise. If the clinician is in doubt about either question, the case should be referred.[6–8]

Three simple questions usually give clinicians a good starting point in allowing patients to express their concerns. These questions are found at the top of the updated January 2015 Smile Evaluation Form (see **Fig. 1B**).

If the clinician has the experience and ability to meet the patient's stated expectations or has a team that can provide the best outcome, careful consideration should then be given to the patient entirely.[8]

This consideration must include a thorough evaluation of the:

1. Facial analysis
2. Occlusion/orthodontic evaluation
3. Phonetic analysis, including swallow evaluation
4. Dentofacial analysis
5. Dental analysis, especially in the smile zone
6. Evaluation of the surrounding hard and soft tissue

Each of these components and how they build on one another provide the lattice structure for the finished case.

Dental photography and/or video recording is becoming more and more the standing operating procedure in this initial consultation visit, because it is often necessary to refer back to these photographs and video to establish a final treatment plan.

The standard set of photographs taken for patients is shown in **Fig. 2**.

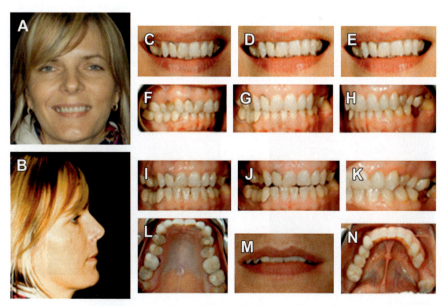

Fig. 2. (*A*) Full-face frontal view. (*B*) Profile view. (*C*) Right smile. (*D*) Centered smile. (*E*) Left smile. (*F*) Right retracted biting. (*G*) Center retracted biting. (*H*) Left retracted biting. (*I*) Right retracted open. (*J*) Center retracted open. (*K*) Left retracted open. (*L*) Maxillary incisal view. (*M*) Rest position. (*N*) Mandibular incisal view.

Collecting these photographs (see **Fig. 2**) a clinician can then superimpose their patients' pictures onto the Smile Evaluation Form. This article now addresses the form so that readers can understand the data collection process and, with practice, may go through the form quickly and accurately. Once accomplished accurately, clinicians can easily glean from this form a good understanding of each patient's needs.

FACIAL ANALYSIS
Frontal View

Facial analysis is checked at a conversational distance. The clinician should visualize and if possible record a series of vertical and horizontal lines to evaluate the existing symmetry of the patient's face. This record will eventually be used to determine the relationship of the patient's face and dentition in space.

The first yellow horizontal line from the top of the figure is called the interpupillary line. It passes through the center of the pupil of each eye (**Fig. 3**). The horizontal line below this is called the commissural line. It passes through the corners of the mouth where the upper and lower lips meet. These lines should normally be parallel to one another and are normally parallel to the anterior dental incisal plane. These landmarks are extremely important in the work of Coachman and Calamita[9] and are used in the new concept of digital dental design. The thickness of the upper and lower lips should be quantified and the patient should be asked about past or planned future lip enhancements or reductions. This information should be noted and referred back to in the future.

The vertical yellow line drawn through the glabella (centered between the eyebrows), the tip of the nose, through the center of the philtrum (just under the nose), through the center of Cupid's bow (the maxillary-facial border of the upper lip), and then to the center of the chin is called the facial midline. This vertical line is important in determining the amount of symmetry in the face. It is generally thought that the more symmetry that exists between the right and left sides of the face, the closer to perfection is the face. Although this perameter is often looked for in professional models, no individuals have a perfectly symmetric face and very few individuals have a face that has close to perfect symmetry. Most dental patients have mild to moderate asymmetry and clinicians should recognize this because it may be necessary to consider this factor in planning the finished restorations (**Figs. 4–7**).

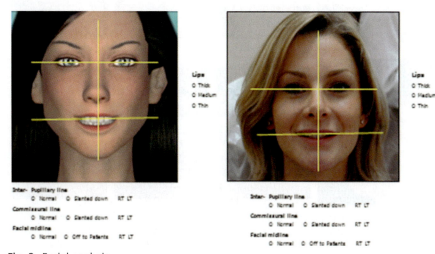

Fig. 3. Facial analysis.

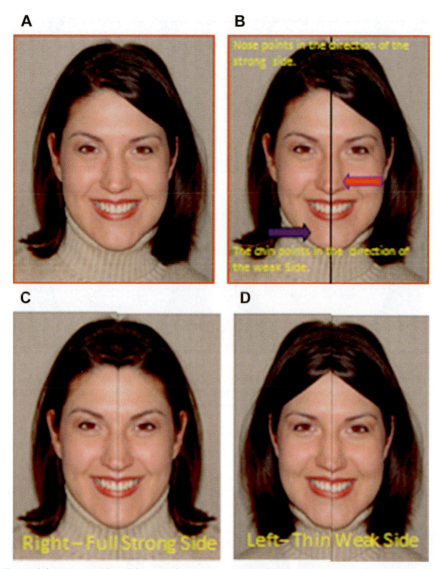

Fig. 4. (*A*) Patient with mild to moderate asymmetry. (*B*) The nose generally points in the direction of the strong side (*the fuller side of the face*), whereas the chin generally points toward the weak side (*the leaner side of the face*). (*C*) Mirror image of the strong side. (*D*) Mirror image of the weak side of the face.

Fig. 7 shows an important imaginary line called the Ricketts E plane. This line, which is drawn from the tip of the nose to the tip of the chin, allows the profile of the patient to be evaluated by comparing the distance from the upper lip to the plane and then the lower lip to the plane. For white men and women, a normal profile has the maxillary lip approximately 2 times the distance to the Ricketts E plane (4 mm) as the lower lip.[9] A concave profile may call for a more prominent position of the maxillary anterior teeth when restoring, whereas a more convex profile may require a less prominent position of the final restorations. Another landmark is called the nasal-labial line angle.

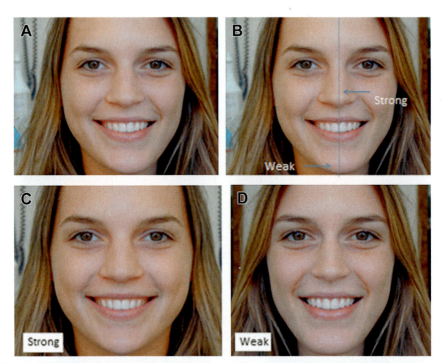

Fig. 5. Mild frontal facial asymmetry. (*A*) Patient, also a professional model, with mild asymmetry. (*B*) The nose generally points in the direction of the strong side of the face, whereas the chin generally points toward the weak side of the face. (*C*) Mirror image of the strong side (*full side*) of the face. (*D*) Mirror image of the weak side (*lean side*) of the face.

Men generally have a 90° to 95° n/l angle, whereas women generally have a 100° to 105° n/l angle.[10]

In **Fig. 8** the face is divided horizontally into 3 almost equal portions. The topmost portion runs from the hairline to the top of the patient's eyebrows. The second portion runs from the eyebrows to the tip of the nose. The lower portion runs from the tip of the nose to the tip of the chin. This third portion is generally slightly wider than the other

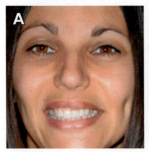
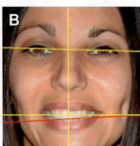
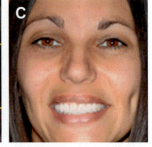

Fig. 6. (*A*) Frontal facial view. The patient's left eye and eyebrow are slightly lower than the right eye and brow. (*B*) A facial midline shows a moderately asymmetrical face. The interpupillary line is slanted down from the patient's right to her left. Her commissural line is parallel to the floor, but her incisal plane is slanted up from her right to her left (*the line in red*). (*C*) A computer-simulated smile was created to predict the final appearance of the restoration, with the caveat that symmetric restorations may not allow a perfect result because of the facial disharmony.

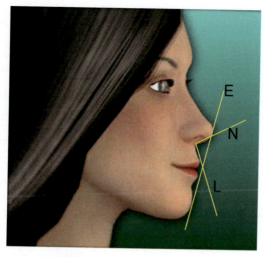

E- plane

O Max ___ mm

O Man ___ mm

Nasal-labial

O > 90 degrees

O < 90 degrees

O = 90 degrees

Profile

O Normal

O Convex

O Concave

Fig. 7. Facial analysis, lateral view. This profile view includes an important imaginary line called the Ricketts E plane. This line drawn from the tip of the nose to the tip of the chin allows the profile of the patient to be evaluated by comparing the distance from the upper lip to the plane and then the lower lip to the plane. See text for more detail.

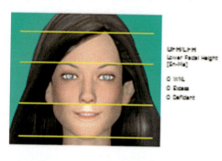

UFH/LFH
Lower Facial Height
[Sn-Me]

O WNL
O Excess
O Deficient

Midline
O Upper and lower midlines coincide with the facial midline
O Upper dental midline is deviated to the   R L   (circle)
O Lower dental midline is deviated to the   R L   (circle)

Overbite
O WNL [0-30%]   O Moderate [31-69%]   O Severe [70-100%]
Anterior Open Bite ___ mm   O Dental   O Skeletal

Overjet
O WNL [1-2 mm]   O Moderate [3-3mm]   O Severe [more than 3mm]

Maxillary		**Mandibular**	
O Crowding	O Spacing	O Crowding	O Spacing
O Anterior Crossbite	O Dental	O Skeletal	O Functional shift
O Posterior Crossbite R or L	O Dental	O Skeletal	O Functional shift

Classification of Occlusion/ Malocclusion
O Normal Occlusion   O CII malocclusion
O CII Div 1   O CII Div 2   O CI

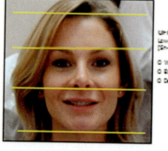

UFH/LFH
Lower Facial Height
[Sn-Me]

O WNL
O Excess
O Deficient

Midline
O Upper and lower midlines coincide with the facial midline
O Upper dental midline is deviated to the   R L   (circle)
O Lower dental midline is deviated to the   R L   (circle)

Overbite
O WNL [0-30%]   O Moderate [31-69%]   O Severe [70-100%]
Anterior Open Bite ___ mm   O Dental   O Skeletal

Overjet
O WNL [1-2 mm]   O Moderate [3-3mm]   O Severe [more than 3mm]

Maxillary		**Mandibular**	
O Crowding	O Spacing	O Crowding	O Spacing
O Anterior Crossbite	O Dental	O Skeletal	O Functional shift
O Posterior Crossbite R or L	O Dental	O Skeletal	O Functional shift

Classification of Occlusion/ Malocclusion
O Normal Occlusion   O CII malocclusion
O CII Div 1   O CII Div 2   O CI

Fig. 8. Occlusion/orthodontic evaluation.

two portions in a youthful patient with no occlusal wear and a normal vertical dimension. However, this portion might shrink with age and severe wear (posterior bite collapse).

The incisal and occlusal analysis is evaluated next (**Fig. 9**) and involves a good history that allows the clinician to diagnose whether or not habits have affected the occlusion, angulations, and buccal-lingual positioning of the teeth. If the clinician does not know the cause of an existing malocclusion/malposition, rebuilding the dentition may be short-lived. Overbite, overjet, space analysis, and classifications of occlusion and malocclusion should be evaluated carefully.

In the 1950s, clinicians came to realize the importance of phonetics in helping to determine denture teeth set-up and appropriate anterior tooth position and length in relation to vertical dimension of occlusion.[11] Patients in physiologic rest position show a space between the upper and lower arch of between 2 to 4 mm.[12] The minimum facial reveal of anterior teeth in this position for a youthful appearance has been identified as between 2 and 4 mm depending on the sex of the individual (women generally show more tooth).[13] The Mmma sound allows a view of the rest position as well as the tooth reveal at this position. This phonetic guide helps in planning the look to be achieved in the initial wax up of a well-planned case (**Fig. 10**). The extended pronunciation of the E sound is another important phonetic guide. This sound provides the widest smile in young individuals. The space between the upper and lower lips should almost completely be filled by the maxillary incisors in pronouncing this sound. The maxillary incise edge is very close to the superior border of the lower lip. As people age, the muscles of the mouth lose tone and less and less of the maxillary teeth are visible during the pronunciation of the long E sound.[14] The S sound is created by air passing between the soft surface of the tongue and the hard surface of the lingual of the maxillary anterior teeth.[15] Correct pronunciation of the F and V sounds is accomplished when the incisal edges of the maxillary anterior teeth make light contact with the lower lip (vermilion border).[16] The incisal edges should be stationed directly over the line of demarcation between the wet and dry border of the lower lip. This mild contact allows a buildup of sufficient pressure for correct pronunciation.

The functional assessment is made during a dental history that includes observations of the patient's swallowing and breathing during the patient interview. A thorough intraoral examination may reveal signs of bruxism and general wear that may indicate incisal and occlusal disharmony. This assessment is also the best opportunity to see whether the facial and dental midlines are coincidental. If the maxillary or mandibular midlines are deviated from the facial midline this should be noted. Canting of the midlines should be noted and diagrammed later in the form. A space analysis should also be categorized and noted (**Figs. 11–13**).

The section shown in **Fig. 14** is extremely important because it allows clinicians to draw directly on the form. Lines can be drawn and labeled to indicate spaces between teeth, overcrowding, poor axial inclination, canting of teeth, areas of existing caries, occlusal interferences, and intrusion or extrusion of teeth. Specific entries available allow clinicians to identify facial contour abnormalities, discrepancy in golden proportion, crown length/width ratio, incisal embrasure abnormalities, inclination problems, tooth spacing, gingival zeniths irregularities, and gingival biotype.

The dental-facial analysis (**Fig. 15**) is a critical component in determining the fine details of designing the restorations that will deliver the eventual esthetics of the case. Identifying the patient's horizontal and vertical components as either normal or needing improvement guides the clinician as to how the case should proceed. The drawings are self-explanatory and after using the form numerous times it can be filled out quickly and accurately with ease. Any component that may require the

Occlusal analysis

Functional assessment

O Digit sucking e.g. thumb   O Lip sucking/biting

O Object biting/sucking   O Mouth breathing

O Tongue thrust swallow   O Clenching

O Grinding / Bruxism   O Other _____

Dental midline

O Upper and lower teeth midlines coincide with the facial midline

O Upper dental midline is deviated to the   **R   L**   (circle)

O Lower dental midline is deviated to the   **R   L**   (circle)

Overbite

O WNL [0-30%]   O Moderate [31-69%]   O Severe [70-100%]

Anterior open bite _____ mm   O Dental   O Skeletal

Overjet

O WNL [1-2 mm]   O Moderate [3-5mm]   O Severe [more than 5mm]

Space analysis

Maxillary

O Crowding   O Spacing (mild, moderate, severe)

Mandibular

O Crowding   O Spacing (mild, moderate, severe)

Fig. 9. Orthodontic evaluation.

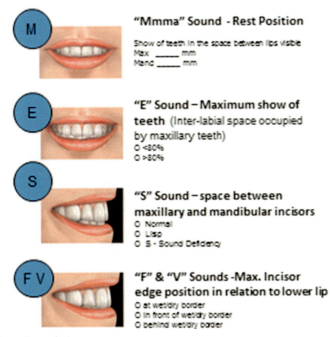

"Mmma" Sound - Rest Position

Show of teeth in the space between lips visible
Max _____ mm
Mand _____ mm

"E" Sound – Maximum show of teeth (Inter-labial space occupied by maxillary teeth)
O <80%
O >80%

"S" Sound – space between maxillary and mandibular incisors
O Normal
O Lisp
O S - Sound Deficiency

"F" & "V" Sounds -Max. Incisor edge position in relation to lower lip
O at wet/dry border
O in front of wet/dry border
O behind wet/dry border

Fig. 10. Phonetic analysis.

consult of another discipline is easily identified and recorded. Understanding the language of esthetics (a topic covered by Dr Nicolas Davis[16]) goes a long way in helping the reader understand the diagrams on the Smile Evaluation Form.

Further explanation of the vertical and horizontal components selected for the updated New York University Smile Evaluation Form are given, using a clinical example, in **Figs. 16–22**.

DISCUSSION

We identified that the patient shown in **Fig. 2** had a lower lip position in which her maxillary anterior teeth incisal edges were touching her lower lip. The canines were in front of the wet/dry border of the lower lip, whereas the centrals and laterals seemed to be on the border. Her lip line showed little, if any, gingival tissue. Her dental midline was offset to the patient's left compared with the facial midline. Kokich and

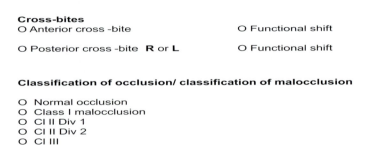

Cross-bites
O Anterior cross -bite   O Functional shift

O Posterior cross -bite **R or L**   O Functional shift

Classification of occlusion/ classification of malocclusion

O Normal occlusion
O Class I malocclusion
O Cl II Div 1
O Cl II Div 2
O Cl III

Fig. 11. A generalized orthodontic evaluation (classification of occlusion or malocclusion is noted).

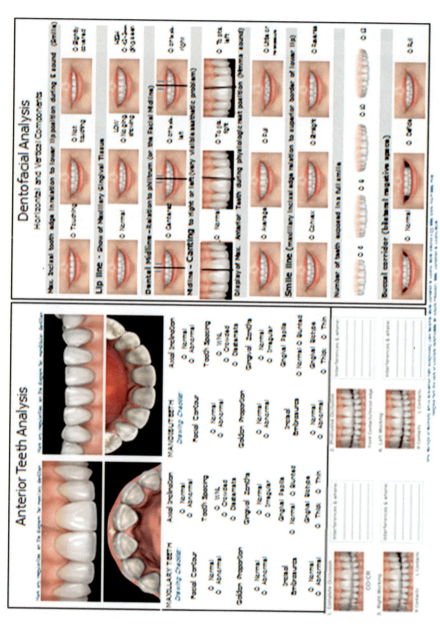

Fig. 12. Smile Evaluation Form (side B), updated January 2015.

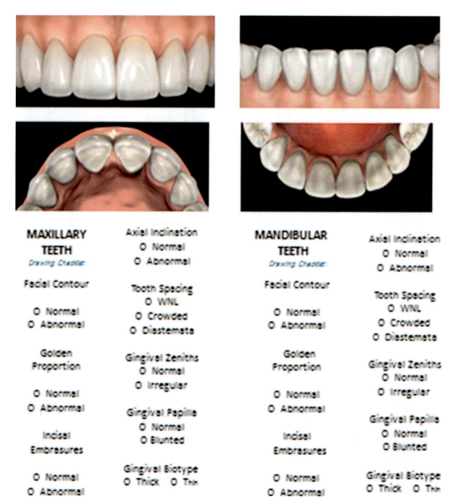

Fig. 13. Anterior teeth analysis; the smile zone.

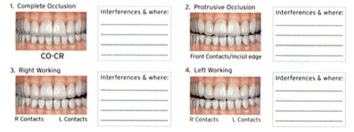

Fig. 14. Occlusion analysis. This important update allows the clinician to record occlusal interferences in centric occlusion (CO), centric relation (CR), protrusive movement, and right and left lateral excursions.

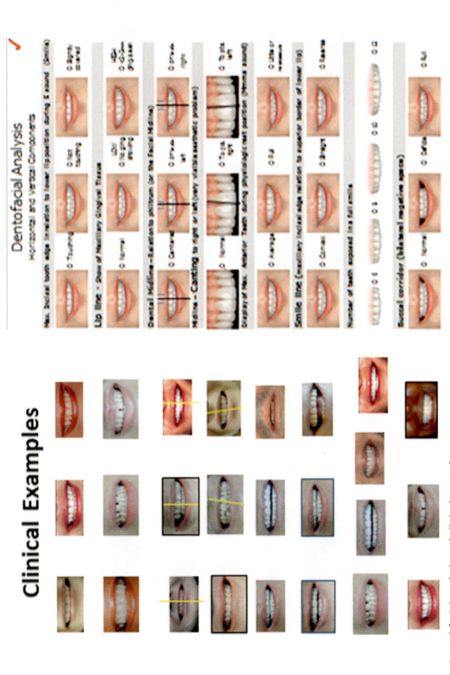

Fig. 15. Dental-facial analysis and clinical examples.

A

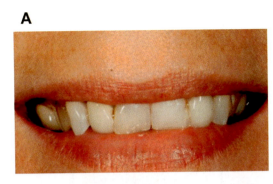

B

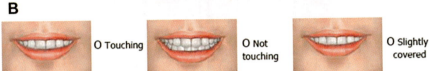

O Touching   O Not touching   O Slightly covered

Fig. 16. (*A, B*) Tooth lower lip position during the pronunciation of the E sound. Provides incisal edge position.

A

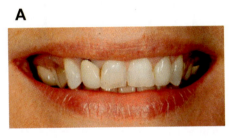

B

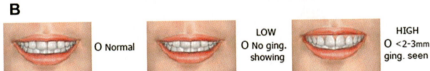

O Normal   LOW O No ging. showing   HIGH O <2-3mm ging. seen

Fig. 17. (*A, B*) Lip line show of maxillary gingival tissue. Ging, gingiva.

A

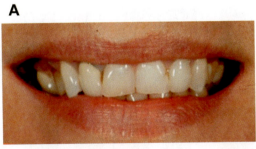

B

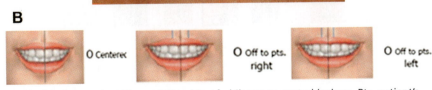

O Centered   O Off to pts. right   O Off to pts. left

Fig. 18. (*A, B*) Dental midline: relationship of philtrum to central incisors. Pts, patient's.

A

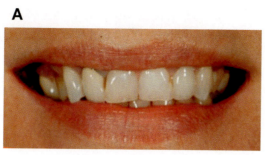

B

| The dental midline is coincidental to facial midline | The dental midline is canted to the patient's right | The dental midline is canted to the patient's left |

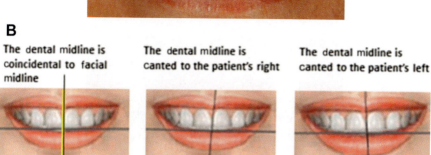

Fig. 19. (*A*, *B*) Midline: canting to right or left.

A

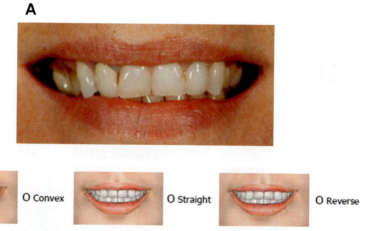

B

O Convex O Straight O Reverse

Fig. 20. (*A*, *B*) Smile line (maximum incisal edge relationship to lower lip).

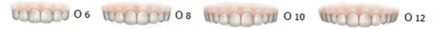

O 6 O 8 O 10 O 12

Fig. 21. Number of teeth exposed in full smile.

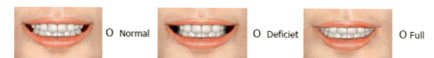

O Normal   O Deficiet   O Full

Fig. 22. Buccal corridor.

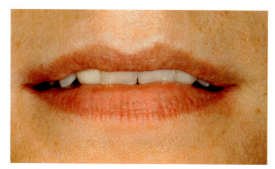

Fig. 23. Patient is at rest pronouncing the Mmma sound.

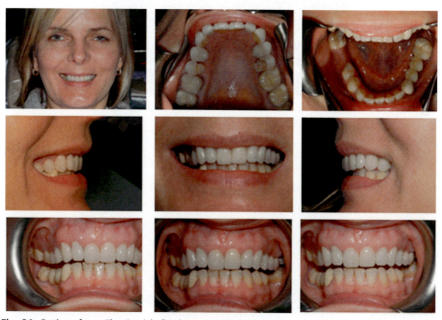

Fig. 24. Patient from **Fig. 2** with final restorations.

colleagues[17] showed that a dental midline can be as much as 3 mm to the right or left of the patent's facial midline and still look aesthetically pleasing, but in this case the dental midline was also canted to the patient's left. This must be addressed in order to achieve an aesthetic result. The display of teeth is 10 when the patient pronounces the E sound but only the front 4 are seen in the Mmma sound (rest position; **Fig. 23**).

This patient showed a straight to reverse smile line and an insufficient buccal corridor. All of these problems are studied carefully to be assured they are addressed in the final restorations. **Fig. 24** shows the patient from **Fig. 2** with final restorations.

SUMMARY

This article updates readers on this simple adjunct to the armamentarium of modern aesthetically minded clinicians. This form is currently in use at New York University College of Dentistry and is now in electronic format (axiUm) as part of the University's decision to go paperless in its record keeping. It will continue to be modified so that more and better information ors can be provided on our patients so the proper treatment planning will be aided. It remains a work in progress and we hope to get feedback on how it can be improved.

ACKNOWLEDGMENTS

The authors acknowledge the pioneering work in smile evaluation forms by Dr Leonard Abrams, Dr Jeffrey Morlry,[3,8] Dr james Eubank,[8] Dr Mauro Fradeani,[13] and Jonathan Levine.[14] We also offer special thanks to our NYU colleagues Drs Jonathan Levine, Sivan Finkel, and Jeffrey McClendon for some of their suggestions in updating the NYU Smile Evaluation Form.

REFERENCES

1. Spear FM, Kokich VG. 2nd edition. A multidisciplinary approach to esthetic dentistry in: successful esthetic and cosmetic dentistry for the modern dental practice, vol. 51. Philadelphia: Dental Clinics of North America, Elsevier; 2007. p. 299–318.
2. Dziezak J. Restoring the ageing dentition. Curr Opin Cosmet Dent 1995;41–4.
3. Morley J. The role of cosmetic dentistry in restoring a youthful appearance. J Am Dent Assoc 1999;130:1166–72.
4. Calamia JR, Levine JB, Lipp M, et al. 2nd edition. Smile design and treatment planning with the help of a comprehensive esthetic evaluation form cosmetic dentistry for the modern dental practice, vol. 51. Philadelphia: Dental Clinics of North America, Elsevier; 2007. p. 188–209.
5. Goldstein RE. Study of the need for esthetics in dentistry. J Prosthet Dent 1969; 21:589–98.
6. Goldstein RE, Lancaster JS. Survey of patient attitudes toward current esthetic procedures. J Prosthet Dent 1984;52:775–80.
7. Feeley RT. Cosmetics and the esthetic patient and laboratory communication. Oral Health 1995;85:9–14.
8. Morley J, Eubank J. Macro-esthetic element of smile design. J Am Dent Assoc 2001;132:39–45.
9. Coachman C, Calamita M. Digital smile design: a tool for treatment planning and communication in esthetic dentistry. QDT 2012 Quintessence 2012;1–9.
10. Kois JC. Diagnostically driven interdisciplinary treatment planning. Seattle Study Club J 2002;6:28–34.

11. Ricketts RM. Planning treatment on the basis of facial pattern and an estimate of its growth. Angle Orthod 1957;27:14–37.
12. Rufenacht CR. Fundamentals of esthetics. Chicago: Quintessence; 1990.
13. Fradeani M. Esthetic rehabilitation in fixed prosthodontics. Vol 1: esthetic analysis: a systemic approach to prosthetic treatment. Chicago: Quintessence; 2004.
14. Levine JB. Esthetic diagnosis in: current concepts in cosmetic dentistry. Quintessence Publishing; 1994. p. 9–17.
15. Pound E. Esthetic dentures and their phonetic values. J Prosthet Dent 1951;2: 98–112.
16. Davis NC. Smile design. Dent Clin North Am 2007;51:299–318.
17. Kokich VO Jr, Kiyak HA, Shapiro PA. Comparing the perception of dentists and lay people to altered dental esthetics. J Esthet Dent 1999;11:311–24.

FURTHER READINGS

Coachman C, Van Dooren E, Gurel G, et al. Smile design: from digital treatment planning. Quintessence; 2012. p. 119–74.
Dawson PE. Restoring upper anterior teeth. In: Dawson PE, editor. Evaluation, diagnosis, and treatment problems. 2nd edition. St Louis (MO): Mosby; 1989.
Dawson PE. Functional occlusion: from TMJ to smile design. St Louis (MO): Mosby; 2007.
Hammond RJ, Beder OE. Increased vertical dimension and speech articulation errors. J Prosthet Dent 1984;52(3):401–6.
Rugh JD, Drago CJ, Barghi N. Comparison of electromyographic and phonetic measurements of vertical rest position [abstract]. J Dent Res 1979;58(Special Issue):316.
Spear FM. Fundamental occlusal therapy of occlusion. Chicago: Quintessence; 1997. p. 421–34.
Spear FM. The maxillary central incisal edge: a key to esthetic and functional treatment planning. Compend Contin Educ Dent 1999;20:512–6.
Vig RG, Brundo GC. The kinetics of anterior tooth display. J Prosthet Dent 1978;39: 502–4.

An Aesthetic and Functional Rehabilitation
A Case Study

Jaafar Ali, DDS, Christine Calamia, DDS, Kenneth S. Magid, DDS*,
John R. Calamia, DMD, Nicholas J. Giannuzzi, DDS

KEYWORDS

- Multidisciplinary treatment • Smile evaluation • Material selection

KEY POINTS

- Gain an appreciation for the complexity of multidisciplinary treatment.
- Realize the indispensable utility of the New York University Smile Evaluation Form.
- Appreciate that an understanding of material properties is critical for long-term success.

PATIENT BACKGROUND AND CHIEF CONCERN

A 48-year-old male owner of a hair salon presented with the chief concern of long, thin, and unaesthetic anterior crowns that hindered his ability to comfortably chew, as a result of several missing posterior teeth. The patient's expectations were to receive a smile makeover and posterior implants that would allow him to function better. He requested a treatment that avoided any orthodontic solutions.

His medical history was unremarkable and noncontributory; thorough extraoral and intraoral examination ruled out any abnormalities of the temporomandibular joint and its associated muscles as well as occlusal disharmonies and parafunctional habits. He had significant dental history that included extensive past fixed prosthodontic and restorative/endodontic therapy.

Clinical examination revealed general failure of restorations throughout the dentition. Teeth numbers 6 to 11 were previously restored with all-ceramic full-coverage restorations.

Teeth numbers 3, 4, 5, 12, 13, 14, 21, and 29 had existing porcelain fused to metal (PFM) crowns. The natural dentition of the mandibular anterior region showed rotation and unevenness with a diastema between teeth numbers 22 and 27. On full smile, there was a significant shade difference between the lower and upper arches. The

NYU College of Dentistry, New York, NY, USA
* Corresponding author. Advanced Dentistry of Westchester, Harrison, NY.
E-mail address: ken.magid@gmail.com

periodontal condition was satisfactory, with probing depths ranging from 1 to 4 mm throughout the maxilla and mandible. Radiographic analysis showed generalized mild horizontal bone loss. No vertical defects, mobility, or fremitus were noted (**Fig. 1**).

A clinical diagnosis was formulated for this patient that included:

- Caries
- Missing and broken teeth with some loss of function
- Generalized mild periodontal disease accompanied by posterior tooth loss
- Right canine class II malocclusion with an anterior open bite
- Moderate crowding in the mandible
- Recurrent lesions around previously endodontically treated teeth with symptomatic apical periodontitis
- Unaesthetic, failing crowns with a significant shade discrepancy from the remaining natural dentition

The goals of the treatment were to control the factors that caused the disease and to restore the deformities that the disease process caused, while achieving an aesthetic outcome acceptable to the patient. A multidisciplinary approach involving fixed prosthetic, periodontal restorative and endodontic therapies was essential to achieving the desired outcome (**Fig. 2A–F**).

SMILE EVALUATION

Pretreatment smile analysis is even more important in patients who have already undergone treatment within the aesthetic zone (**Fig. 3**).

A step-by-step approach to this analysis was achieved using the New York University (NYU) Smile Evaluation Form (Forms 1 and 2), from which the information obtained was communicated to the dental technician for the fabrication of a full-mouth diagnostic wax-up (see **Fig. 3**).

Facial analysis revealed normal lips, an interpupillary line that was canted down to the patient's right compared with the intercommisural line, and a symmetric facial midline that corresponded with the maxillary dental midline.

Occlusal and orthodontic evaluation (**Fig. 4**) revealed a lower dental midline that was 4 mm to the right of the upper midline. Facial thirds were symmetric, a flat facial profile was noted with the upper lip 6 mm and the lower lip 5 mm behind the Ricketts E-plane.

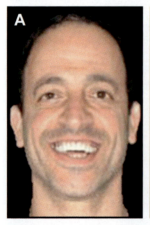
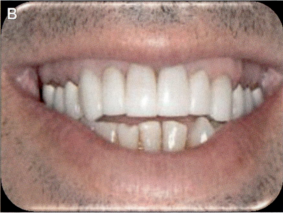

Fig. 1. (*A, B*) A 48-year-old patient presents with unaesthetic and failing crowns, reverse smile line, anterior open bite, lower arch crowding, and missing teeth causing a functional loss.

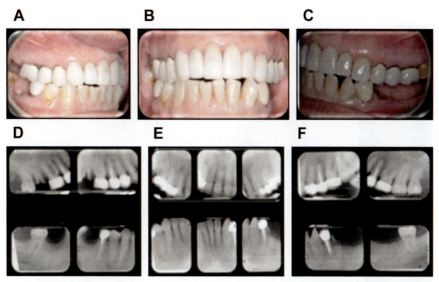

Fig. 2. Preoperative right (*A*), frontal (*B*), and left (*C*) lateral retracted views of the patient in maximum intercuspation. Note the narrow width of the anterior maxillary crowns, open bite, open margins in posterior full coverage restorations, exaggerated Curve of Spee, rotated mandibular left canine with moderate anterior crowding, and shade difference between the upper and lower dentition. (*D–F*) A series of radiographs showing mild horizontal bone loss; nonrestorable teeth, some with residual periapical disorder and large screw-retained posts; overprepared maxillary anterior teeth under all-ceramic full coverage restorations; and missing and traumatized teeth.

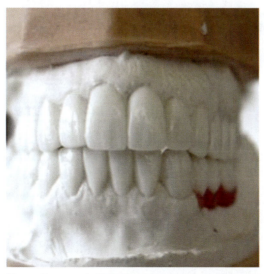

Fig. 3. Full-mouth diagnostic wax-up. Note the closure of the anterior open bite and correction of the reverse smile line was achieved by lengthening numbers 7,8,9,10. Proper positioning and definition of the line angles on these teeth allowed us to fabricate restorations that did not appear longer than at initial presentation. Also note that, at initial planning, the correction of the occlusal plane posteriorly might necessitate the use of pink porcelain in the final PFM implant crown restorations.

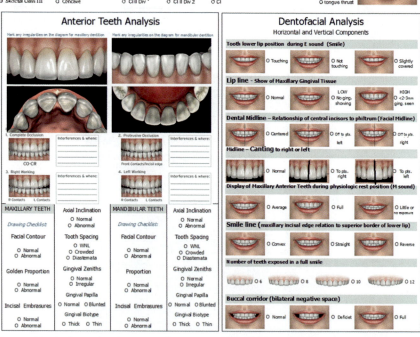

Fig. 4. NYU Smile Evaluation Form. (*Courtesy of* [NYU College of Dentistry Smile Evaluation Form] John Calamia, DMD, Jonathan B. Levine, DMD, Mitchell Lipp, DDS; and *Adapted from* the work of Leonard Abrams, 255 South Seventeenth Street, Philadelphia, PA 19103, 1987; Dr Mauro Fradeani, Esthetic Rehabilitation in Fixed Prosthodontics, Quintessence Publishing, Carol Stream, IL, 2004; and Jonathan B. Levine, DMD, GoSMILE Aesthetics, 923 5th Avenue, New York, NY 10021.)

The nasolabial angle was slightly acute. A right canine class II and left canine class I relationship existed under a skeletal class I base with mild to moderate crowding in the mandible and an anterior open bite. The patient showed a right posterior crossbite.

Phonetic analysis (see **Fig. 4**) with the E sound revealed a reverse smile line with 100% of maxillary teeth and 30% of mandibular teeth occupying the interlabial space within a full buccal corridor. No lisp was detected with the S sound and the upper incisal edges met frontal to the wet/dry border of the lower lip on F.

With 5 mm of interdental space, 10% of the upper and lower anterior teeth were displayed on the M sound. Examination of the anterior dentition (**Figs. 1, 2**, and **4**) revealed abnormal gingival and facial contours of the maxillary teeth with nonideal embrasure spaces and axial inclinations. Although no significant deviation from the Golden percentage was noted, there was a significant width/height discrepancy. A considerable amount of thick keratinized gingival tissue was noted in the maxilla and mandible, especially in the aesthetic zone, with some localized areas of recession in the posterior regions.

A step-by-step approach to this analysis was achieved using the NYU Smile Evaluation Form.

TREATMENT PLANNING

Generating a successful treatment plan necessitates meticulous collection of information and proper integration of these data to formulate a correct diagnosis. Delivering a treatment plan to achieve a final restoration that would predictably reestablish the patients function and simultaneously deliver a highly aesthetic outcome was challenging.

With regard to the open bite, reverse smile line, and small width/height ratios of the anterior maxillary crowns, options to successfully correct these abnormalities were contemplated as follows:

- Should orthodontic extrusion of the premaxilla and/or intrusion of the posterior maxillary segments be considered to correct the exaggerated Curve of Spee and gumminess of the posterior segments? Respecting the patient's wishes to avoid orthodontic therapy made this modality of correcting the deformities inacceptable.
- If orthodontic therapy is not an option, can the anterior open bite be restoratively eliminated without making the teeth appear even longer than they already do? Although this is was probably the only option left to correct the open bite, it was imperative that detailed instructions regarding the shape, size, and contours of the relevant teeth and the position and definition of the central and lateral incisors' line angles be communicated to the ceramist before fabrication of the final restorations.
- In an attempt to further eliminate the appearance of a negative smile line, is bilateral maxillary crown lengthening necessary to reduce the excessive display of gingiva in the posterior segments? The final treatment did not require osseous surgery; the gingival recession in these areas was sufficient to allow us to place the margins of the new restorations more apically and correct the occlusal plane accordingly.
- A multidisciplinary treatment plan was developed for the patient and sequenced as follows:
  - Initial periodontal therapy, including scaling and root planning of 4 quadrants.
  - Caries restoration on teeth numbers 15 and 17 and retreatment of failed endodontic therapy on tooth 6.
  - Extraction and socket preservation at sites 2, 3, 4, 20, and 21. Tooth number 13 was extracted and immediately temporized for development of an ovate pontic site (**Fig. 5**).

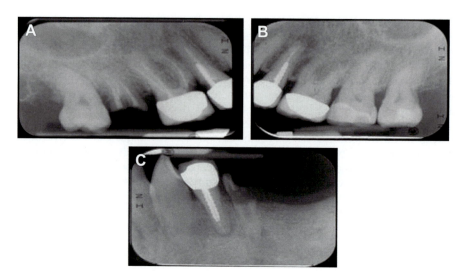

Fig. 5. (A–C) Periapical views showing radiographic evidence for nonrestorability of teeth 2, 3, 4, 13, 20, and 21. Note that all teeth had undergone prior endodontic treatment, and that half of them were restored using large screw-retained posts and showed signs of persistent periapical disorder.

- Ridge augmentation at edentulous area of tooth 30.
- Two-stage implant placement at teeth numbers 3, 4, 18, 20, 21, and 30.
- E-max crowns at teeth numbers 5 to 11, 22, and 29; 3 unit Lava fixed partial denture (FPD) numbers 12 to 14, and veneers 22 to 28. Definitive restorations of implants using PFM crowns.
- Occlusal guard and 3-month recare interval.

TREATMENT SEQUENCE
Phase I: Preventative

Because of the significant dental history, it was imperative that the patient be properly instructed to establish adequate oral hygiene and be motivated to commit to the maintenance of his final restorations. Visual cues (ie, demonstration of flossing) were used to educate the patient on the importance of home care. After initial therapy was performed, the patient was prescribed Prevident 5000 Plus and placed on a 3-month periodontal maintenance and recare interval.

Phase II: Eradication of Disease and Development of Sites for Implant Placement

Teeth numbers 15 and 17 were restored on the occlusal and mesial-occlusal surfaces, respectively, using composite. The right maxillary canine was endodontically treated because of a persistent periapical radiolucency and symptomatic apical periodontitis.

Fig. 4 shows nonrestorable teeth (numbers 2, 3, and 20). Numbers 4, 13, and 21 had residual disorder after insufficient endodontic treatment and restoration with large screw-retained posts. Because of the poor prognosis of retreatment, these teeth were also treatment planned for extraction. Each of the extraction sites except number 13 were rinsed thoroughly and packed with mixed irradiated human cortical and cancellous allograft (Rocky Mountain Tissue Bank) over which a nonresorbable membrane (Osteogenics Cytoplast) was secured with a horizontal mattress suture.

The grafted sites were allowed to heal for a period of 3 to 4 months.

Clinical examination and analysis of the cone-beam computed tomography (CBCT) data revealed an alveolar height and width deficiency in the edentulous area of tooth number 30. This lack of native bone required ridge augmentation to achieve the necessary hard tissue profile for implant placement. A full-thickness midalveolar incision was made taking extra care to preserve the keratinized tissue. Two vertical releasing incisions were made at the distofacial line angle of teeth numbers 28 and 31, were extended just past the mucogingival junction, and the flap released. The buccal bone was decorticated and Exactech Regenaform RT Allograft Paste mixed with clindamycin was placed on buccal bone. Two screws were used to tent a Geistlich Bio-Guide membrane placed over the graft and 3.0 Vicryl sutures were placed to achieve primary closure of the site.

Phase III: Restoration of Oral Function and Aesthetics

1. Implant placement at sites 3, 4, 18, 20, 21, and 30.

    Dental implants are quickly becoming the restoration of choice for the replacement of missing teeth. Precise evaluation of the hard and soft tissue morphologies and an understanding of the limitations of implant placement are key to a successful outcome (**Fig. 6**).

    CBCT is the gold standard for precise implant planning, especially in larger reconstructive cases. Three-dimensional implant positioning software (Simplant software, Materialize Dental; Glen Burnie, MD) was used to strategize the implant placements.

    Sizes of implants were chosen according to the amount of bone available at each site. Surgical stents were fabricated with a plastic matrix.

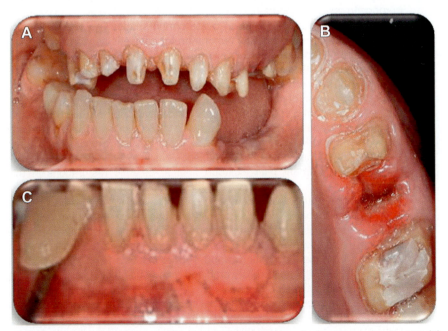

Fig. 6. (*A*) Preparation of the maxillary teeth. (*B*) Development of ovate pontic site #13. (*C*) Preparation for mandibular veneers; a shade taken.

Sites 3, 4: cantilever temporaries 4 to 5 were removed. An incision was made distal to number 5 and a flap raised. Two Superline Dentium implants (4.3 × 10 mm) were placed at the sites. Cover screws were secured and primary closure achieved with 3.0 silk sutures.

2. Sites 19, 20, and 21: after reviewing the computed tomography (CT) scan, it was noted that the mental foramen was located in the ideal site for the 19 implant. The decision was made to place the implant further distal to avoid the foramen. Incision was made distal to 22. Superline Dentium implants placed at sites 19 (3.8 × 8 mm), 20 (3.4 × 8 mm), and 21 (3.4 × 10 mm). All cover screws were placed and 3.0 sutures were placed to achieve primary closure.

3. Site 30: the locations of the existing screws were noted in the CT scan. A midcrestal incision was made with 2 vertical releases. One Superline Dentium implant (3.8 × 10 mm) was placed at site. A cover screw was placed and primary closure achieved with 3.0 silk sutures. A provisional was fabricated using a matrix fabricated over the diagnostic wax-up, which was filled with the temporary crown material Luxatemp (DMG America; Englewood, NJ). This prototype temporary was seated for 1 minute and 45 seconds then quickly removed; it showed evidence of minimal tooth structure remaining under the patients existing maxillary restorations. Tooth 13 was extracted before careful removal of all maxillary full-coverage restorations. Underlying caries were excavated and immediately restored with nanohybrid composite (TPH Spectrum, Caulk/DENSTPLY). The preparations were minimally refined to ensure readable margins and adequate restorative space for the final restoration. A putty matrix, fabricated from the diagnostic wax-up, was filled with temporary crown material (Luxatemp, DMG America; Englewood, NJ) to create a provisional restoration. This prototype temporary was seated for 1 minute and 45 seconds, then quickly removed and reseated over the preparations to allow for a final set of the material.

The fully cured provisional was then removed, trimmed, and polished. Flowable composite resin was bonded to the intaglio surface of number 13 to mold the tissue at the extraction site to an ovate pontic shape. The patient was instructed evaluate the temporary restoration for aesthetic concerns.

4. Mandibular preparations and anterior guidance.

Correcting the esthetics and function in the mandibular anterior region was challenged by the problems of severe rotation of number 22, 4-mm midline shift, the moderate crowding of numbers 23 to 27, and anterior open bite. Several factors were considered in deciding how to restoratively manage the treatment:

- The teeth needed to be restored for a satisfactory esthetic outcome regardless of whether orthodontics was performed. With 30% of mandibular anterior teeth showing in the E smile and the patient's desire to avoid orthodontic intervention, the treatment plan included final all-ceramic restorations in this region.

- The occlusion could be managed with restorative dentistry. In an effort to address the concern of closing the open bite and establish anterior guidance with canine disclusion without compromising the esthetic outcome, a Luxatemp provisional was fabricated over unprepared teeth 22 to 29 using a stint fabricated from the diagnostic wax-up. Proper occlusion and ideal esthetics were confirmed with the maxillary arch and mandibular teeth before preparing lower teeth for final restorations.

- Structural compromises were minimal to correct the malalignment. When correcting anterior crowding without orthodontics, restorative dentists have to find a balance between achieving appropriate reduction without compromising the biological constraint of maintaining pulpal vitality. Derotation of tooth 22 was achieved by preparing the tooth for a full-coverage ceramic restoration without the need for a prophylactic endodontic treatment. The use of buccal and incisal indices (Reprosil putty, Dentsply/Caulk; Milford, DE) guided the preparations of the remaining mandibular teeth in ideal positions to alleviate the crowding and achieve functionally sound esthetic restorations. Teeth 22 to 28 were reduced with modifications to the ideal veneer preparation. Number 29 was prepared to be restored with a full coverage after crown lengthening and fabrication of a new post and core.

5. Material selection and final restorations.

Proper understanding of the restorative material limitations and requirements for success in a complex oral environment are key to long-term clinical success. A rationale for material selection was developed using the guidelines discussed in the review article by McLaren and Whiteman. Our decision to use 4 different categories of materials for the final restorations for this patient concurred with the investigators' philosophy that a "restorative material and technique should be chosen to allow the most conservative treatment that will satisfy the patients esthetic, structural and biological requirements while having the mechanical properties to provide clinical durability".

Materials were selected based on 6 clinical parameters as outlined by the investigators:

- Space required for color change
- Esthetics
- Substrate
- Flexure risk assessment
- Excessive shear and tensile strength assessment
- Risk of bond failure

Feldspathic Porcelain Veneers for Teeth 23, 24, 25, 26, 27, and 28

With the exception of the rotated mandibular left canine, the mandibular anterior teeth and first bicuspid were reduced to an average depth of 0.5 mm, leaving more than 80% of the substrate and greater than 90% of the margin in enamel. Conservative reduction of this amount of tooth structure provided sufficient space for color change and allowed high-strength bonding to the porcelain, thus greatly reducing the risk of flexure and bond failure of these restorations. The shallow overbite, lack of unsupported porcelain, and absence of parafunctional habits decreased the risk of tensile and shear stresses.

IPS e.max Full-Contoured Crowns Over Teeth 5, 6, 7, 8, 9, 10, 11, and 29

Because of prior reduction of the maxillary dentition, substrate condition was not in accordance with the authors' recommendation for using glass ceramic materials (**Figs. 7** and **8**). However, monolithic IPS e.Max was still used as the material of choice for these restorations as it demonstrates high esthetics and possess a low flexure risk and medium risk of failure due to debonding and tensile and shear stresses.

Veneered Lava Zirconia Core for FPD 12-X-14

Although esthetics was not of primary concern in this high-stress area, sufficient reduction of at least 1.5 mm was provided for the core and veneering porcelain. The core design of the FPD functions as a stable substrate for powder/liquid porcelain, especially in situations of minimal enamel, and provides added support for this area of high flexure risk and unfavorable stress distribution.

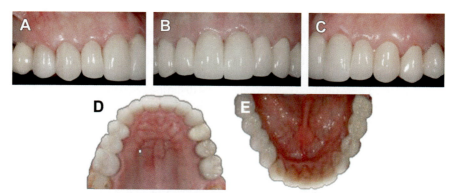

Fig. 7. (*A*) Maxillary right quadrant implants in teeth 3 and 4 restored with PFM crowns. (*B*) Canine–to-canine view of the tooth 5 to 11 E-max crowns. (*C*) Maxillary left quadrant lava bridge of teeth 12 to 14. (*D*) Maxillary occlusal view of the ceramic restorations mentioned earlier. (*E*) Mandibular occlusal view including feldspathic porcelain veneers on teeth 22 to 28 and implants on teeth 18, X, 20, 21, and 30 with E-max crowns.

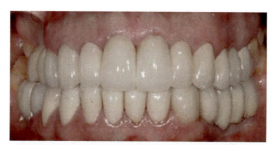

Fig. 8. Retracted frontal view of the final rehabilitation. Note the healthy tissue profile, better width/length ratio of the maxillary centrals, and closed anterior open bite.

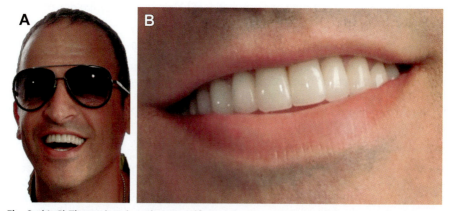

Fig. 9. (*A*, *B*) The patient is no longer self-conscientious about his smile and, on the contrary, is confident about his natural appearance.

Porcelain Fused to Metal for Implant Crowns Number 3, 4, 18, 19, 20, and 30

Proper planning of the implant positions using the information obtained from the CBCT and diagnostic wax-up was critical in avoiding the need for custom abutments when restoring the implants. Ceramometal restorations have been the gold standard of full-coverage restorations for more than a half-century and were the ideal choice of material for final implant crowns (**Fig. 9**).

SUMMARY

This article describes a multidisciplinary approach to a functional and esthetic rehabilitation. We were able to successfully close the anterior open bite and correct an exaggerated Curve of Spee restoratively while still maintaining a highly esthetic outcome. The maxillary anterior teeth no longer appear to have a disproportional width/length ratio and are in better balance with the mandibular veneers. Functional compromise was reestablished, mostly with implant retained crowns. Occlusal harmony and stability are maintained by cuspid guidance and anterior disclusion of posterior teeth in protrusive. Proper selection of the final restorative material is imperative for the long-term survival of the restorations.

ACKNOWLEDGMENTS

Special thanks to Oleg Gorlenko (CDT) of Americus NY-Dental Services Group, 163-15 Hillside Ave, Jamaica, New York, for his excellent laboratory work in the rehabilitation of this patient.

RECOMMENDED READINGS

Culp L, McLaren EA. Lithium disilicate: the restorative material of multiple options. Compend Contin Educ Dent 2010;31(9):716–20, 722, 724–5.

Fahl N Jr, McLaren EA, Margeas RC. Monolithic vs. layered restorations: considerations for achieving the optimum result. Compend Contin Educ Dent 2014; 35(2):78–9, 20.

Giordano R. A comparison of all ceramic systems. J Mass Dent Soc 2002;50(4): 16–20.

McLaren EA, Cao PT. Ceramics in dentistry—part I: classes of materials. Inside Dent 2009;5(9):94–103.

McLaren EA, Cao PT. Smile analysis and esthetic design: "in the zone". Inside Dent 2009;5(7):44–8.

McLaren EA, Rifkin R. Ceramics: rationale for material selection. Compend Contin Educ Dent 2010;31(9):666–8, 670.

McLaren EA, Whiteman YY. Treatment selection for anterior endodontically involved teeth. Pract Proced Aesthet Dent 2004;16(8):553–60.

Rifkin R, McLaren E. Macroesthetics: facial and dentofacial analysis. J Calif Dent Assoc 2002;30(11):839–46.

Sadowsky SJ. An overview of treatment considerations for esthetic restorations: a review of the literature. J Prosthet Dent 2006;96(6):433–42.

Replacement of Old Porcelain-Fused-to-Metal Crowns and Smile Rejuvenation Using All-Ceramic Restorations

Kateryna Grytsenko, DDS, John R. Calamia, DMD, FAGD*

KEYWORDS

- Rehabilitation • Veneers • Monolithic onlay • All-ceramic crowns

KEY POINTS

- Previous restoration failure is recognized.
- The probable cause of these failures is determined.
- Decision is made regarding the new treatment plan and sequence of treatment.
- Treatment is provided, and results are observed.
- The plan for maintenance is charted.

PATIENT BACKGROUND

A 29-year old woman presented to the New York University College of Dentistry (NYUCD) clinic for a possible replacement of her old broken restorations and for possible Invisalign (Align Technology, Inc, San Jose, CA) treatment. Her chief complaint was "I want my lower and upper teeth to match in color and alignment" (**Fig. 1**). The patient reported extensive restorative and prosthodontics treatment of her upper arch 15 years ago in Russia. She mentioned that she liked how crowns matched her natural teeth in the beginning, but as time went by and "all her friends got whiter teeth by means of veneers or bleaching," she started to want to get rid of the yellow hue in her teeth (**Fig. 2**). Apart from that, the patient started noticing the chipping of her lower front teeth and one of the crowns on the upper teeth (**Fig. 3**). The crowding of the lower front teeth had always been a concern of the patient; however, she was hesitant to do anything about it because she wanted to avoid extensive preparation of those teeth, as had happened on the upper teeth (see **Fig. 3**). The

The authors have nothing to disclose.
* Corresponding author.
E-mail address: jrc1@nyu.edu

Dent Clin N Am 59 (2015) 559–569
http://dx.doi.org/10.1016/j.cden.2015.03.012
0011-8532/15/$ – see front matter © 2015 Elsevier Inc. All rights reserved.

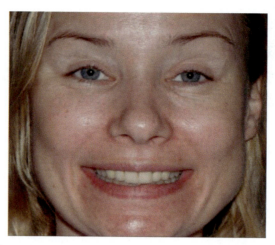

Fig. 1. Initial visit.

patient also mentioned that she might have needed a couple of old fillings replaced (**Figs. 4** and **5**). The patient was eager to change the restorations and start the treatment, but she did not want it to be "too invasive." Her primary concern was esthetics, but she did not want any long all-embracing treatment.

Medical history was noncontributory; the patient reported no drug allergies.

DIAGNOSTICS AND TREATMENT PLAN

Extensive diagnostic methods were used to analyze the intraoral situation. Full-mouth series of radiographs, panoramic radiograph, and diagnostic casts with wax-up were completed and investigated. Smile analysis form was filled out to determine the guidelines for ideal esthetics of the future restorations (see **Fig. 3**; **Fig. 6**).[1]

At the time of the examination, teeth #6 to #11 had porcelain-fused-to-metal crowns with metal lingual surfaces and chipped incisal edge on teeth #10 and #11 (see **Figs. 2–5**). Crowns on teeth #6 to #11 were splinted for no apparent reason (**Fig. 7**). Periodontal probing was difficult in the area because of deep subgingival margins of the restorations and significant bleeding on probing. Intraoral examination also revealed deep bite, crowding, and enamel wear of the lower anterior teeth (see **Figs. 2–5**).

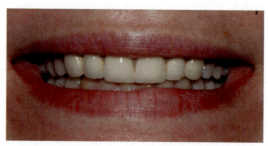

Fig. 2. Close-up smile.

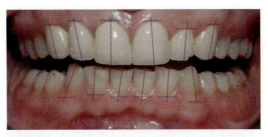

Fig. 3. Dental analysis.

Periodontal status of the rest of the dentition was within normal limits. Tooth #8 had periapical radiolucency. According to the patient, the root canal in tooth #8 was completed 15 years ago and never really bothered her (see **Fig. 7**). Tooth #12 had a big distal-occlusal restoration; the tooth was vital and asymptomatic. Tooth #13 had a root canal retreatment completed at postgraduate clinic 1 month ago and required further post, core, and full-contour restoration. Tooth #16 had deep caries on the buccal surface, a class 5 lesion. Tooth #17 was partially erupted with frictional keratosis in the area of operculum. Tooth #21 had recurrent decay under the distal-occlusal restoration (see **Fig. 7**). Tooth #32 was supraerupted. The patient noted she sometimes clenches her teeth.

After thorough diagnostics and consultations with orthodontist, periodontist, and prosthodontist, it was suggested to the patient to proceed with full-mouth rehabilitation involving orthodontics and full coverage restorations on the posterior teeth. She declined the ideal treatment plan and emphasized her only esthetic concern. So, it was decided to include teeth #4 to #13 and teeth #22 to #27 in the following alternative treatment plan:

- Extract teeth #16, #17, and #32.
- Section and remove teeth #6 to #11, refine preparations.
- Prepare teeth #4 and #5, #22 to #27 for veneers.
- Prepare teeth #12 and #13 for full coverage crowns.
- Perform gingivectomy on teeth #22 to #27 using diode laser.

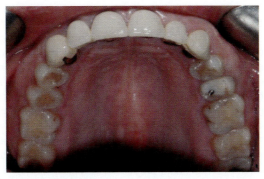

Fig. 4. Occlusal view of maxillary arch.

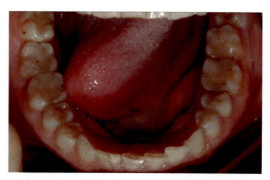

Fig. 5. Occlusal view of mandibular arch.

- Perform apicoectomy of tooth #8.
- Composite restoration of tooth #21 DO (Distal/occlusal surfaces of the tooth), class 5 buccal, #20 class 5 buccal.

Maxillary right first and second premolars were included in the plan owing to display of teeth when smiling (see **Fig. 1**). It was also explained to the patient that root canal retreatment could be completed on tooth #8 before working on crowns. But the patient opted to rather go for apicoectomy if the tooth becomes symptomatic after the restorations would have been changed. Teeth #20 and #21 as well as #28 and #29 were initially planned for veneers, but eventually it was decided to use in-office bleaching to achieve desirable color and bond the class 5 lesions with composite where necessary, thus, preserving the tooth structure, as per patient's concern.

TREATMENT

Teeth #16, #17, and #32 were extracted 1 to 2 months before start of the treatment without any postoperative complications.

Crowns #6 to #11 were sectioned using diamond and carbide burs. Teeth #22 to #27 were prepared for veneers (**Figs. 8** and **9**). Preparations were refined, and provisional restorations were fabricated using bisacryl. Polyvinyl-siloxane material (light and medium body) was used for final impressions (**Fig. 10**). B1 was selected as the final restoration color. Because of extensive black discoloration of teeth #7 and #8, it was particularly challenging to match the color of the final restorations. Stump shades were determined, and the photographs sent to the laboratory with final impressions and instructions (**Figs. 11** and **12**). The discoloration also influenced the choice of material for final restorations. In-office bleaching was completed for the lower arch to enhance the color matching of maxillary and mandibular restoration. On removal of old crowns from teeth #6 to #11, it was discovered that clinical crowns were short and no additional incisal reduction could have been done. At the same time, it was necessary to block the dark shade of the underlying tooth structure. So, a thin and strong material was chosen for crowns on teeth #6 to #13, Lava Zirconia Crowns (3M ESPE).[2] Diode laser gingivectomy was completed for lower anterior teeth to create more even gingival zeniths and increase the clinical crown lengths, without extensive surgical involvement.[3] Final restorations were fabricated from feldspathic porcelain for teeth #4 and #5 as well as #22 to #27 and zirconia copings with feldspathic veneering for teeth #6 to #13. Permanent restorations for teeth #6 to #13 were cemented using resin-modified glass ionomer (RMGI) cement, and all veneers were cemented

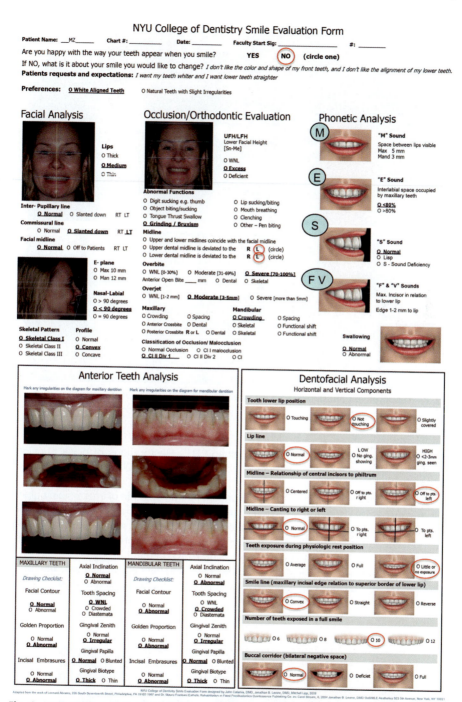

Fig. 6. NYU College of Dentistry smile evaluation form. (*Courtesy of* John Calamia, DMD; Mitchell Lipp, DDS; and Jonathan B. Levine, DMD; *Adapted from* Leonard Abrams, 255 South Seventeenth Street, Philadelphia, PA 19103, 1987; and Dr Mauro Fradeani, Esthetic Rehabilitation in Fixed Prosthodontics Quintessence Publishing Co, Inc, Carol Stream, IL, 2004.)

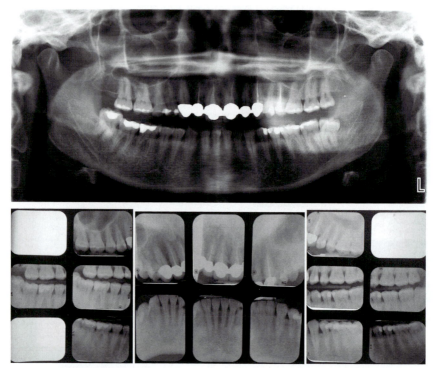

Fig. 7. Preoperative panoramic radiograph and full-mouth series of radiographs.

permanently using flowable composite (shade B1). Restorations of class 5 lesions were done using composite material (shade B1) on teeth #20 and #21. Night guard was fabricated.

During the course of the treatment, the patient had an episode of irreversible pulpitis in tooth #30. Root canal therapy (RCT) was completed in the undergraduate clinic at NYUCD with no postoperative complications (**Fig. 13**). Because the clinical crown of the tooth was short, it was decided to fabricate the full contour restoration from mono-lithic zirconia.[2] The crown was cemented using RMGI cement.

The patient was very satisfied with the final result and her new smile (**Figs. 14–19**). In fact, right after taking the final 1-week follow-up pictures, she asked whether

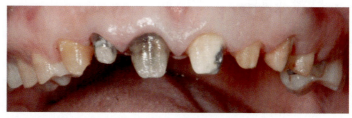

Fig. 8. Veneer and crown preparations for teeth #4 to #13.

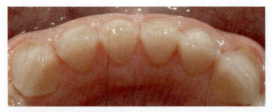

Fig. 9. Teeth #22 to #27 veneer preparations.

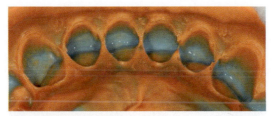

Fig. 10. Teeth #22 to #27 final impression.

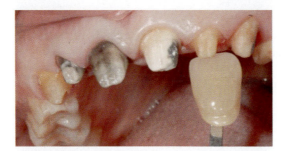

Fig. 11. Stump shade for maxillary restorations.

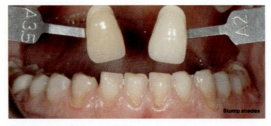

Fig. 12. Stump shade selection for mandibular restorations.

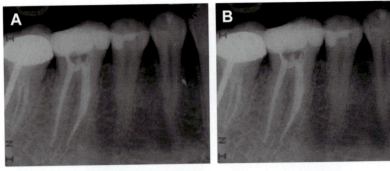

Fig. 13. (*A*, *B*) Completed RCT of tooth #30.

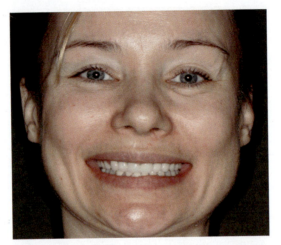

Fig. 14. Postoperative full face smile.

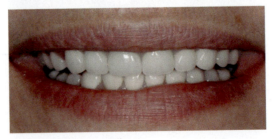

Fig. 15. The day of insertion close-up smile.

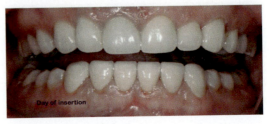

Fig. 16. The day of insertion, retracted view.

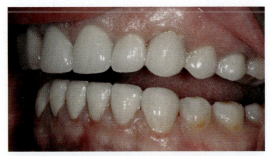

Fig. 17. The day of insertion, close-up left side.

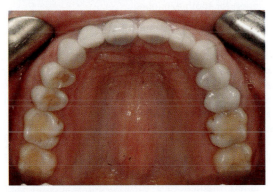

Fig. 18. Postoperative maxillary occlusal view.

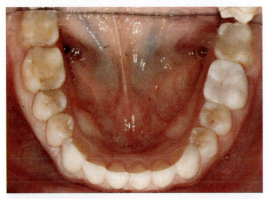

Fig. 19. Postoperative mandibular occlusal view.

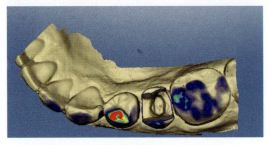

Fig. 20. CAD/CAM impression scan for tooth #20.

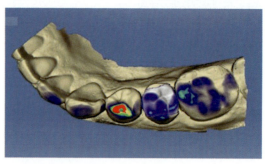

Fig. 21. CAD/CAM design for tooth #20 inlay.

something could be done with her old fillings in the lower left. Tooth #19 DO and mesial occlusal (MO) and tooth #20 DO were placed a while ago. The teeth were asymptomatic, but the patient noted that sometimes she gets food stuck in between. On clinical examination, poorly contoured direct composite restorations with poor marginal integrity were discovered. It was explained to the patient that desirable outcomes could have been achieved with full-contour crowns or inlay/onlay type of restorations. She opted for onlays to preserve as much tooth structure as possible. On preparation of teeth #19 and #20, the buccal pulp horn of #20 was exposed and RCT was recommended. Tooth #19 was completed at the same appointment using computer aided design/computer aided manufacture (CAD/CAM) unit with Blue-Cam and Vita Empress block shade A1. Perfect color match was achieved for tooth #19. The onlay was cemented using dual-cure cement. On completion of RCT in the undergraduate clinic, inlay in tooth #20 was completed using the same technology, but a different shade (B1) was used as per the patient's request. It is worth mentioning that the patient was using the at-home bleaching gel only until the first and second premolars on the lower arch. Therefore, there was a color discrepancy in the final onlay and inlay restorations; B1 blended perfectly with bleached tooth #20 and A1 matched the natural color of tooth #19 (**Figs. 20–22**).

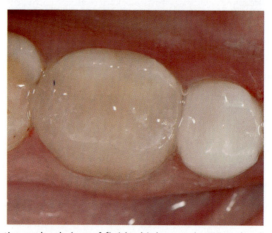

Fig. 22. Postoperative occlusal view of finished inlay tooth #20 and onlay tooth #19.

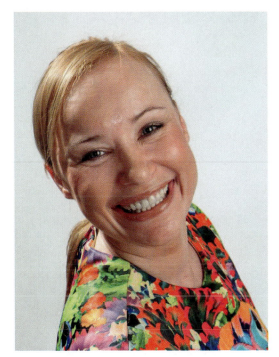

Fig. 23. Two months postoperation.

SUMMARY

An interdisciplinary approach and multiple types of materials were used because of the complexity of this case. The choice of materials was based on evidence-based literature search, current occlusal scheme, desirable aesthetic outcome, and core technique of the university.

A highly desirable result and complete patient satisfaction was achieved (**Fig. 23**).

ACKNOWLEDGMENTS

Special thanks to Dr K.S. Magid, DDS; Dr N. Giannuzzi, DDS; and Dr F.A. Puccio for their guidance in this case.

REFERENCES

1. Calamia JR. Successful esthetic and cosmetic dentistry for the modern dental practice. Dent Clin North Am 2007;51(2):281–571.
2. Bachhav CC. Zirconia-based fixed partial dentures: a clinical review. Quintessence Int 2011;42(2):173–82.
3. Lee EA. Laser- assisted crown lengthening procedures in the esthetic zone: contemporary guidelines and techniques. J Contemp Esthetics 2007;42–9.

Restoration of the Dentition in a Patient with a History of Non-Hodgkin Lymphoma and Gastroesophageal Reflux Disease

Manila Nuchhe Pradhan, DDS, John R. Calamia, DMD*

KEYWORDS

- GERD • Ceramic restoration • Laser crown lengthening • Undergraduate training

KEY POINTS

- Today's dental patients are concerned about dental disease and their appearance.
- Clinicians often must decide not only the type of restoration, but also the material used for restoration to provide aesthetics and longevity.
- A modern practitioner should know the pros and cons of different types of crowns and veneers with regard to survival, success rate, and aesthetic result.
- Clinicians also provide treatment for patients with complicated medical histories; risk assessments include current conditions, risks of recurrence, and suggestions for future maintenance of restorations.

PATIENT BACKGROUND

A 42-year-old Hispanic man presented to the New York University (NYU) College of Dentistry for the first time in April of 2009. The patient's chief concern was the appearance of his anterior teeth. He presents with spacing between maxillary anterior teeth, which were small and worn down. He is a married man with 2 children and happy with his personal life. He works as an accountant.

SOCIAL HISTORY

- History of use of alcohol (≤2 drinks each day but stopped 13 years ago).
- History of tobacco use (one-half a pack of cigarettes a day but stopped 4 years ago).

Disclosures: None.
* Corresponding author.
E-mail address: jrc1@nyu.edu

Dent Clin N Am 59 (2015) 571–582
http://dx.doi.org/10.1016/j.cden.2015.03.015   **dental.theclinics.com**

MEDICAL HISTORY

- Review showed that he had a history of non-hodgkin lymphoma diagnosed in 2007, which was a diffused B-cell–type lymphoma, present around kidney, ureter, and in the bone marrow. He underwent intravenous chemotherapy from April to September 2007.

  He went for follow-up every 3 months after the chemotherapy through January 2009 and had a good recovery with no relapse. After January 2009, he has been going for 6-month follow-up visits, and is considered to be in remission. He no longer takes any medication for the disease.
- The patient also has a history of gastroesophageal reflux disease (GERD), for which he has been prescribed esomeprazole (Nexium) by his physician. Currently, he is not taking any other medications.
- His vital signs are with in normal limit with blood pressure of 115/80, pulse of 68, and respiratory rate of 16.
- Family history is remarkable for hypertension (HTN) and diabetes, but no history of any kind of cancer.

DENTAL HISTORY

- He used to go to a private dentist but found it too expensive and came to NYU in 2009 as the result of a referral from one of his friends.
- Most of his private care was minor restorations (fillings) and adult prophylaxis.
- He was a compliant regular patient and has continued to be compliant at NYU.
- He states he brushes once a day but never flosses.
- He also volunteered that he grinds his teeth at night.

He did shown concern about his teeth color. His extraoral soft tissue examination was within normal limits with no enlargement of lymph nodes.

His chief complaint (CC) is: "I am not very happy with my front teeth, which has wide spaces, they are chipped and I want to do something about it." He did receive consults for orthodontics and prosthodontics, but could not afford the postgraduate fees. In September of 2011, the patient was referred to the undergraduate Honors Aesthetics Clinic for an aesthetics consult and workup.

INITIAL ORTHODONTIC VISIT

The patient's orthodontic template from when he presented initially is provided in **Fig. 1**.

RADIOGRAPHIC EXAMINATION

Intraoral soft tissue examination was within normal limits (**Fig. 2**). Intraoral hard tissue examination showed generalized moderate periodontitis with significant bone loss. Probing depths ranged from 3 to 4 mm on anterior and posterior teeth. All third molars had been extracted. Generalized spacing around teeth 4, 5, 6, 7, 8, 9, 10, 11, and 12 was noted.

Existing Restorations Included

#3- Occlusal amalgam restoration
#18- Occlusal amalgam restoration
#19- Occlusal buccal amalgam restoration
#30- Occlusal buccal amalgam

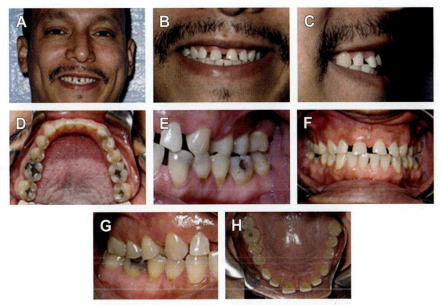

Fig. 1. Orthodontic template of patient when he presented. (*A*) Preoperative full face. (*B*) Preoperative smile. (*C*) Preoperative right lateral view. (*D*) Preoperative mandibular occlusal view. (*E*) Preoperative retracted left lateral view. (*F*) Preoperative retracted frontal view. (*G*) Preoperative retracted right lateral view. (*H*) Maxillary incisal view.

#31- Occlusal amalgam

All existing amalgam restorations were rated acceptable and without secondary decay; #29 showed an E2 distal lesion, which was kept under observation. He was prescribed Prevident 5000 plus. Calculus was noted on lower posteriors 18, 29, 30, and 31.

The patient presented with concerns about the spacing in his anterior teeth, as mentioned. Clinically, the facial profile was straight, with spacing in maxillary arch. Both the right and left molar and canine relationships were recorded as a class II. The overbite was about 1 mm and he exhibited close to an edge-to-edge relationship. When the patient was referred, he had already gone through an orthodontic evaluation

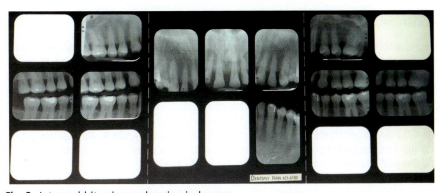

Fig. 2. Intraoral bitewing and peri-apical x-rays.

and postgraduate prosthodontic consult, then esthetic treatment to enhance esthetics. The occlusion as far as patient could remember had been like that, but he said that he had noticed more spacing in front over the years and the tooth had worn a lot. When inquired about his habit he said that when he was young he used to suck on lemons a lot. He was diagnosed with GERD during his early adulthood and he had grinding habit.

Problem list
- Moderate periodontitis
- Spacing on anterior maxillary teeth; a problem owing to patient's concern

Risk Assessment

Caries risk
Patient was put under high caries risk owing to E2 calcification that was seen on distal of #29.

Periodontal risk
Generalized plaque and calculus retention around most anterior and posterior teeth with prior loss of attachment was noted. There was no mobility or furcation involvement on any teeth. He was not taking any medication nor did he have any systemic condition that increased his periodontal risk to high. There were no mechanical overhangs or crowding and the probing depths were all less than 4 mm. The patient was rated as moderate periodontal risk.

Cancer risk
Patient has a history of non-hodgkin lymphoma, which was diagnosed in 2007 and treated with intravenous chemotherapy. He is currently considered to be in remission. Because he has a positive history for a previous cancer, he is under high cancer risk. His soft tissue examination was within normal limits. There were no lymphadenopathy and he will be under close surveillance. He is followed every 6 months medically for his lymphoma. His last laboratory values were normal and done 3 months ago. He was a smoker with history of one-half a pack a day for 10 years, but he quit smoking 4 years ago as of 2009. He was moderate alcohol user but stopped 13 years ago, with 1 to 2 glasses a day for the 8 to 10 years he was using it.

Nutrition
When asked about his dietary habits, he said that he balanced it with good amount of green vegetable and protein and tried to stay away from fast food. He drinks 2 cups of coffee a day, and is quite fond of soda.

HEALTH PROMOTION PLAN

Mr J is a 42-year-old Hispanic man who reports a history of drinking 2 or fewer glasses of alcohol each day, but stopped 13 years ago. He used to smoke about one-half a pack of cigarettes a day, but stopped 4 years ago. He has a family history of HTN and diabetes. His vitals were within normal limits (blood pressure, 115/80 mm Hg; pulse, 68; respirations, 16). His body mass index was 26.6 kg/m^2, which is slightly overweight (normal range, 18.5–24.5). He works as an accountant and has sedentary work but mentions that he tries to exercise at least 3 times a week. As mentioned, he has high caries and moderate periodontal risk but has a very high cancer risk. He is regular with his dental checkup of every 6 to 8 weeks.

Nutrition counseling was to be done to encourage his healthy eating habits and balance between protein, vegetables, and fruits. Because he mentioned his fondness to soda, which explains the tooth erosion owing to acid, it should be explained to the patient about the consequence of it and encourage him to cut down and eventually replace it with water. With his body mass index of 26.6 kg/m^2, he is at high risk for HTN, but he states that he maintains an active lifestyle.

Prevident 5000 plus was also to be prescribed owing to his E2 lesion and minimal intervention (MI) paste to be given owing to his habit of acidic food consumption.

Oral hygiene instructions were also to be given, and explained to the patient that the attachment loss that was seen was owing to a lack of a proper hygiene routine. Use of a motorized tooth brush is recommended. Proper flossing and brushing has to be taught. He seems pretty regular with dental visit, which should be encouraged.

His family history is remarkable HTN and diabetes, which is a risk factor for him, so awareness about it and possible effect of it to the oral health has to be stressed.

According to Taylor and Borgnakke,[1] evidence reviewed supports diabetes as having an adverse effect on periodontal health and periodontal infection having an adverse effect on glycemic control and incidence of diabetes complications.

This patient is at very high cancer risk because he has had non-hodgkin lymphoma in 2007 and underwent chemotherapy. He is aware of his risk and he goes for his recall/recare every 6 months to his general practitioner. Evidence suggests his risk of secondary malignancy.

Our findings suggest that differing immunologic alterations, treatments (eg, alkylating agent chemotherapy), genetic susceptibilities, and other risk factors (eg, viral infections, tobacco use) among lymphoma subtypes contribute to the patterns of second malignancy risk.[2]

TREATMENT PLAN
Phase 1

Oral hygiene instruction, nutrition counseling, taking impression for study cast and preoperative pictures, and radiographs, followed by detailed oral evaluation and comprehensive care plan.

Phase 2

Scaling and root planing of all 4 quadrants need to be done. Scaling and root planing is known to change a gram-negative bacterial population to a gram-positive population. It smooths the root surface, making the surface area more biocompatible for reattachment and formation of long junctional epithelium and it cleans out necrotic cementum. Patient to be given oral hygiene instruction, proper brushing and flossing technique to be shown and reinforced at every visit.

Phase 3

Orthodontics consultation
Prosthetics consultation
Aesthetic consultation—treatment

Phase 4

Occlusal guard

Phase 5

Recare every 3 months

TREATMENT PROVIDED IN SEQUENCE

2/14/11 - Detailed oral evaluation done. Prevident prescription given.

2/28/11- 4BW and 3 Ps taken. Interpretation done. Treatment plan done.

3/10/11- LRQ SRP done, OHI given.

4/08/11- SRP URQ done. OHI given.

4/18/11- SRP ULQ and LLQ done OHI given.

5/06/11- 4–8 weeks reevaluation for periodontal treatment done. Patient was referred to Aesthetic Program for consultation.

9/23/11- Initial Undergraduate Aesthetic Program Consultation examination was begun. Careful attention was given to understand the patient's dental concerns as well as his aesthetic concerns.

A Smile Evaluation Form was filled out (**Fig. 3**).

The Initial Smile Evaluation confirmed much of what had been discussed previously, but it identified the many aesthetic problems present and provided the clinician with a good picture of what needed to be addressed to satisfy the patient's needs functionally, physiologically, and aesthetically.[3]

09/30/11 AESTHETIC TREATMENT –FIRST VISIT

- Esthetic smile evaluation from gone over with the faculty to determine if other adjuncts may be necessary to formulate a sound treatment plan.
- Probing of all upper anterior and the premolars was accomplished to see how the previous periodontal therapy and oral hygiene instruction had done in promoting a better periodontal foundation for planned restorative work. Special attention was paid to the facial gingival readings because laser correction of the gingival zeniths was being considered.
- Additional photos were taken to conform with the basic views necessary in the clinician's presentation of this case to the other members of the program as well as the consulting faculty.
- Two sets of alginate impressions were a taken making sure to transfer the facial midline to the impression tray, which is then transferred to the eventual poured cast. This is the starting point to establish a dental midline that is coincidental with the patient's facial midline. The patient was dismissed for the day while the clinician poured up the casts. One set was kept as a baseline model and the second cast was articulated and a diagnostic wax up begun.

Wax up was done (**Fig. 4**), taking into consideration the patient's existing occlusion. The total width from the mesial of the first premolar to first premolar was measured and the golden proportion used to determine the approximate widths of each tooth, canines, centrals, and laterals. The centrals were begun first with the mesial surface starting at our facial midline as recorded on the cast and the distal margin estimate on dividing the total width from first premolar to first premolar. Once the MD width is determined the length is adjusted to the 8 to 10 ratio of the width to the length usually found in the central incisors.

Over the next 4 weeks, the clinician will develop a treatment plan sequence that she will present to her fellow program participants and the program faculty. By doing this, the input of the whole program is used in determining the best course of treatment for this patient (**Fig. 5**).

VISIT 2: 11/11/11

Treatment plan was presented.

Empress crowns on # 6, #7, #8, #9, #10, and #11 were chosen. The erosion on lingual surface, and lack of enamel prompted a full coverage restoration.

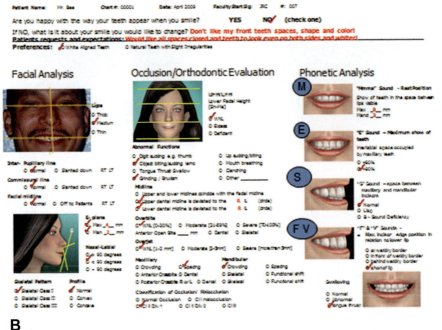

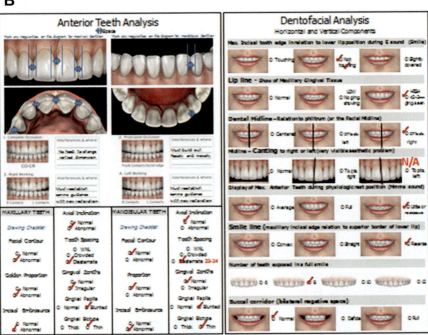

Fig. 3. (*A*) Completed New York University (NYU) smile evaluation form. (*B*) Anterior teeth analysis and dentofacial analysis on NYU smile form. (*Courtesy of* John Calamia, DMD; Mitchell Lipp, DDS; and Jonathan B. Levine, DMD, GoSMILE Aesthetics, 923 5th Avenue, New York, NY 10021; Adapted from Leonard Abrams, 255 South Seventeenth Street, Philadelphia, PA 19103, 1987; and Dr Mauro Fradeani, Esthetic Rehabilitation in Fixed Prosthodontics Quintessence Publishing Co, Inc, Carol Stream, IL, 2004.)

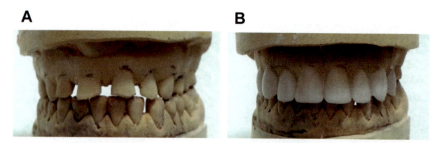

Fig. 4. (A) Original study model. (B) Study model after diagnostic wax-up.

Empress three-quarters veneers on #5 and #12 were chosen to conserve tooth structure, because full coverage would have called for minimum reduction of 2 mm at shoulder and occlusal. However the upper anterior incisors need soft tissue diode laser gingivaplasty, which was explained to the patient to gain 1.5 mm of length for the incisors and harmonize the gingival zenith.

Enameloplasty on lower anterior was done to gain adequate clearance.

A 2-year clinical evaluation of IPS Empress Restorations (Ivoclar Vivadent, Lichtenstein), showed a 100% success rate for crowns[4] in a comparison of IPS Emax and Procera, IPS Emax has superior translucency but not as good strength. Procera is known to have crack propagation and with this patient's history of bruxism Empress 2 was selected.

Patient agreed on the treatment and a mock-up was done on the same visit to show him how he might look.

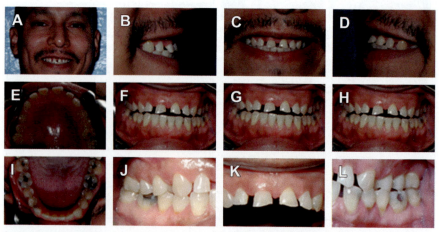

Fig. 5. Preoperative series of photos for patient. (A) Preoperative full face smile. (B) Preoperative right lateral view. (C) Preoperative full frontal view. (D) Preoperative left lateral view. (E) Maxillary incisal palatal view. (F) Preoperative retracted right lateral view. (G) Preoperative retracted frontal view. (H) Preoperative retracted left lateral view. (I) Mandibular incisal view. (J) Preoperative retracted right lateral view, close up. (K) Preoperative retracted frontal view, close up. (L) Preoperative retracted left lateral view, close up.

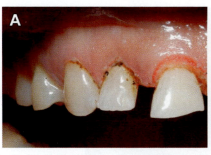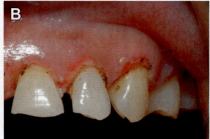

Fig. 6. (*A, B*) Diode laser gingivaplasty done.

VISIT 3: 12/02/11

Bleaching chairside Zoom and at home kit was given.

VISIT 4: 12/09/11

Diode laser gingivaplasty on #6, #7, #8, #9, #10, and #11 was done (**Fig. 6**).

Crown preparation on #6 through #11 and temporized with Luxatemp. Note the gingival margin healing. Crown prepared and temporized (**Fig. 7**).

VISIT 5: 1/13 /12

Three-quarters veneer preparation on #5 and # 12 done.

Existing temp removed preparation from #6 through #11 refined. Final impression taken. Temporized with Luxatemp again (**Fig. 8**).

VISIT 6: 1/27/12

All temporary crowns were removed. After numbing the patient, all the crowns and veneers were placed in order and tried in with a drop of water. Patient was satisfied with the shade and the esthetics.

All crowns and veneers were removed and cleaned. It was well-dried with air. A drop of Silane coupling agent was placed in each crown. The prepared tooth were pumiced, and then etched with phosphoric acid. Optibond Solo Plus was placed on tooth. After

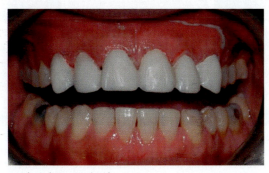

Fig. 7. Crown prepared and temporized.

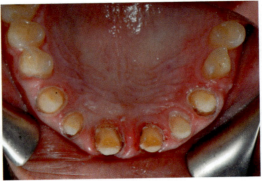

Fig. 8. All the preparations. Note the three-quarters facial veneer preparation on #5 and #12.

that, each crown that had a shade of A1 was filled with resin of same shade and cemented one by one by spot curing and making sure all excess was removed and contact was obtained. Choice 2 light cured cement (Bisco Dental Co, Schaumburg, IL) was used even though the crowns averaged 1.5 mm thick. It was decided that 30 seconds of light curing on both the facial and lingual surfaces would be more than enough to cure the resin cement (**Fig. 9**).

ASSESSMENT: OUTCOME OF CARE AND PROGNOSIS

The treatment given followed the treatment plan. Most of the treatment was based on addressing the patient's chief concern related to esthetics. Risk assessment done related to caries, periodontal health, and cancer was reinforced every visit. Patient was asked about his brushing habit, his use of Prevident and MI paste. Patient's oral hygiene was good. After completion of the treatment, it was noticed that patient was very enthusiastic to maintain his new smile and overall health of oral cavity. The patient will be called in every 3 months for periodic examination going forward. The

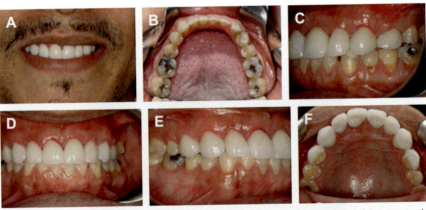

Fig. 9. Template right after cementation of crowns and porcelain veneers. (*A*) Postoperative smile. (*B*) Postoperative mandibular incisal view. (*C*) Postoperative retracted left lateral view. (*D*) Postoperative retracted frontal view. (*E*) Postoperative retracted right lateral view. (*F*) Postoperative mallary incisal view.

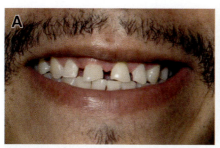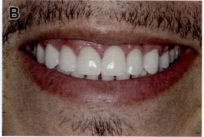

Fig. 10. (*A*) Smile before treatment. (*B*) Smile after treatment.

patient is also reminded to go for his 3-month visit with his physician and keep his medical history updated with necessary blood work every time he comes for his dental workup and screening for oral cancer is done regularly.

With the treatment that has been given, a risk factor had been controlled—patient education is a key element to reducing risk and creating awareness about caries and the relationship with dietary habits. Periodontal health and risk factors were explained and shown in radiographs. It was no surprise that with his investment to getting a beautiful smile, he is very keen on brushing, flossing, and periodic cleaning.

The prognosis of treatment seems very good in long run, because the treatment followed scientific studies, patient's awareness seems very high, and he follows up regularly with his clinician. This treatment took longer than 9 month because this case had to be worked up in different department and could only be done every other Fridays.

SUMMARY

The outcome of the treatment was, in the patient's words, amazing (**Figs. 10–12**). The patient received the best treatment to address his concerns. The risk factors were constantly kept in mind. It was a life-changing experience for him. After 2 weeks of trying out the restorations with no concerns about occlusion reported, the patient came back for impressions for an occlusal guard. Good oral hygiene, occlusal guard, use of MI paste, regular follow-up every 3 months, and patient compliance are key to the success of this treatment in the long run. Treatment planning is an part of dentistry. The patient's concern should be addressed in the treatment planning and at the same time they should be made aware of limitations in dentistry. The success of any

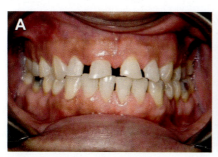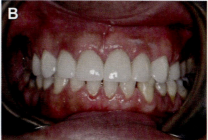

Fig. 11. (*A*) Retracted smile before treatment. (*B*) Retracted smile after treatment.

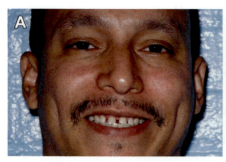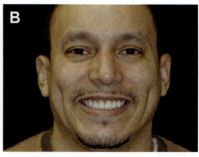

Fig. 12. (*A*) Preoperative photograph. (*B*) Postoperative photograph.

treatment depends on the patient's awareness, compliance, and proper planning, which both the dentist and the patient must understand.

ACKNOWLEDGMENTS

Special thanks to Dr Kenneth Magid for his help and aid in laser surgery needed in this case and Mr Bhaskar Joshi, for picture editing.

REFERENCES

1. Taylor G, Borgnakke W. Periodontal disease: associations with diabetes, glycemic control and complications. Oral Dis 2008;14:191–203.
2. Morton LM, Curtis RE, Linet MS, et al. Second malignancy risks after non-Hodgkin's lymphoma and chronic lymphocytic leukemia: differences by lymphoma subtype. J Clin Oncol 2010;28:4935–44.
3. Calamia JR, Levine JB, Lipp M, et al. Smile design and treatment planning with the help of a comprehensive esthetic evaluation form. Dent Clin North Am 2007;51(2): 187–209, vii.
4. Etman MK, Woolford MJ. Three-year clinical evaluation of two ceramic crown systems: a preliminary study. J Prosthet Dent 2010;103(2):80–90.

Restoration of Fluorosis Stained Teeth: A Case Study

Barbara Slaska, DDS[a], Arnold I. Liebman, DDS[b],*, Diana Kukleris, DDS[c]

KEYWORDS

- Fluorosis • Golden proportion • Teeth-whitening • Porcelain veneer restorations

KEY POINTS

- Dental fluorosis manifests itself by too much ingestion of fluoride resulting in disturbances in enamel mineralization.
- The result is an intrinsic discoloration in the maxillary and mandibular teeth with a poor esthetic appearance.
- In challenging cases, an esthetic result may be achieved only by a combination of techniques.

The patient was a 35-year-old African American man originally from Senegal, Africa who presented to New York University College of Dentistry with the chief complaint of discoloration of his anterior teeth and the desire to have white natural-looking and straight teeth (**Figs. 1** and **2**). His chief complaint: "I need cosmetic work."

MEDICAL HISTORY

There was no significant medical history.

DENTAL HISTORY

A full mouth series of radiographs were taken that displayed no carious lesions. Diagnostic casts were made and the American Academy of Cosmetic Dentistry series of photographs were taken. Teeth #14, #19, and #30 were missing. A dental implant was proposed for future placement in the #30 position. The space was too narrow in the other positions. A class I malocclusion with bimaxillary protrusion was present.

The authors have nothing to disclose.
[a] Department of Cariology and Comprehensive Care, New York University College of Dentistry, 77 East 12th Street, New York, NY 10016, USA; [b] Department of Cariology and Comprehensive Care, New York University College of Dentistry, 2280 East 71st Street, New York, NY 11234, USA; [c] Private Practice, 1248 Farm to Market 78, Schertz, TX 78154, USA
* Corresponding author.
E-mail address: smiledentist3@gmail.com

Dent Clin N Am 59 (2015) 583–591
http://dx.doi.org/10.1016/j.cden.2015.03.003
0011-8532/15/$ – see front matter © 2015 Elsevier Inc. All rights reserved.

dental.theclinics.com

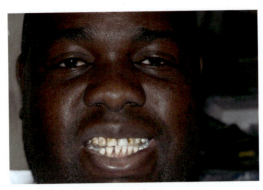

Fig. 1. Full-face view of severe anterior fluorosis case.

This condition is characterized by protrusive and proclined upper and lower incisors and an increased procumbency of the lips.[1]

A New York University College of Dentistry Smile Evaluation Form was completed. A clinical examination was performed and the basic restorative work subsequently completed. Periodontal examination revealed the need for scaling and root planing to achieve desired gingival health. The periodontal status showed local and generalized recession. Periodontal probing and charting revealed sulcus depth was within normal limits but mild gingivitis was present.

TREATMENT PLAN AND SEQUENCING

The patient's esthetic problem was caused by fluorosis. Treatment options included bleaching; microabrasion; direct or indirect composite resin; porcelain veneers; and all ceramic crowns, such as e.max (Ivoclar Vivadent, Amherst, NY) with some opacity to mask the discoloration but still allow an esthetic restoration by combining an opaque core with an esthetic veneer of feldspathic porcelain. The conservative treatment of bleaching in conjunction with feldspathic veneers was selected.

PROGNOSIS

The depth of the staining could not be ascertained. Teeth bleaching was used to reduce the discoloration of the teeth before preparation and therefore the necessity for more opaque veneers. This would allow a more natural appearance of the final veneered teeth and allowing for an excellent prognosis.

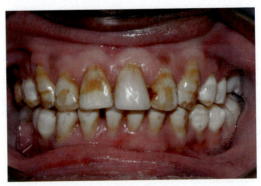

Fig. 2. Retracted view of severe anterior fluorosis case.

TREATMENT SEQUENCING
Periodontal Considerations

Scaling and root planing resulted in the resolution of the patient's gingivitis. A healthy periodontium created the appropriate environment for the restorative phase of treatment. The gingival zeniths were determined to be in the correct position and no surgical intervention was required.

Restorative Considerations

The initial phase requires in-office bleaching (Philips Zoom Light-Activated Whitening System [Philips Oral Healthcare, Stamford, CT]). An initial shade was taken to document the change (see **Fig. 2**; and **Fig. 3**). Three bleaching sessions were performed with 15-minute cycles in the same visit (**Figs. 4** and **5**).

Feldspathic porcelain veneers on eight upper teeth were suggested subsequent to the bleaching. However, financial constraints permitted only teeth #6 to #11 to be treated. Bleaching was performed on the lower arch to improve their appearance and an acceptable result was accomplished. The concept of golden proportion without any spacing was used to guide the wax-up and mock-up before preparation for the porcelain veneers.

The preparations were done with a diamond chamfer bur and guided with a preparation guide to have a controlled reduction (**Fig. 6**). The stains were taken out when prepared with a 0.5-mm facial reduction. In this case the staining was not deep, although unknown before preparation. If the staining was deeper, a deeper preparation would have been required.

Final impressions were taken with Dentsply Reprosil polyvinyl siloxane (Dentsply Caulk, Milford, DE) and the resulting stone model was evaluated for adequate preparation. Provisionals were created from the wax-up using Luxatemp Shade A-1 (DMG America, Englewood, NJ), which was placed into a putty matrix.

The laboratory was supplied with the study models of the wax-up. Feldspathic porcelain was used for the veneers to obtain the most esthetic result. Opaque porcelain was ordered to block-out the discoloration of the color of the teeth.

When the case came back it was placed onto the model to check for accuracy before the patient's appointment **Fig. 7**.

The etched restorations were silanated with Bis-Silane (Bisco, Schaumburg, IL) (**Fig. 8**) and Bisco Choice 2 bonding agent was placed and light cured. Bisco Choice 2 resin cement shade translucent was used as the luting cement. This cement is a high

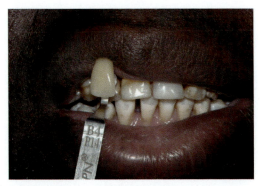

Fig. 3. Initial shade taken to document shade change.

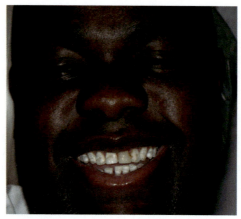

Fig. 4. Result of teeth bleaching.

compressive strength, light-cured luting cement designed specifically for cementation of porcelain and indirect composite veneers (**Fig. 9**).

DISCUSSION

Dental fluorosis is caused by too much ingestion of fluoride resulting in disturbances in enamel mineralization. This results in an intrinsic discoloration in the upper and lower teeth causing a poor esthetic appearance.

The extent of severity depends on the length, term, and quantity of fluoride overexposure. There exist a variety of additional factors that further influence the risk and susceptibility to developing dental fluorosis. Among these are age, growth, weight, and nutrition of the individual.[2–5] The risk for developing fluorosis begins at 3 months and ends at 8 years of age. Once the tooth has erupted, it is no longer at risk for developing this condition.

It is well known that the addition of artificial fluoride to drinking water has numerous benefits in dental caries prevention.[6] Recent studies indicate overexposure to fluoride in some regions of the world, such as Africa, India, and China, where ongoing endemics of systemic fluorosis result from overexposure to naturally occurring fluoride ingested through water.[7–9]

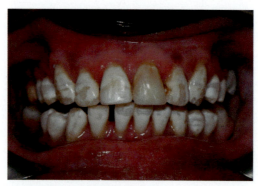

Fig. 5. Retracted view of result of teeth bleaching.

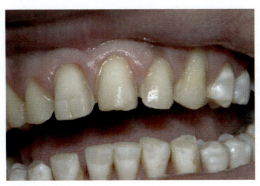

Fig. 6. Veneer preparation showing stains removed.

To best assess the severity and treatment of dental fluorosis, one may refer to the Thylstrup and Fejerskov index.[10] One may also use the fluorosis diagnosis index by Dean, largely known for determining the optimal fluoride concentration (1 ppm) in drinking water.[11–13] Dean categorized mild fluorosis as small opaque areas or streaks covering less than 25% of the tooth surface, moderate as showing brown staining and wear on the occlusal surfaces, and severe as affecting all teeth causing mottling in addition to brown staining.[14,15]

Having dental fluorosis further affects the individual psychosocially. Such individuals report embarrassment to smile, have difficulties pursuing relationships, and lack self-esteem.[16] Furthermore, having fluorosis is perceived as unesthetic and as having poor oral hygiene.[16,17] Dental restorative procedures improve the overall esthetics and may result in increased psychosocial confidence in such individuals.

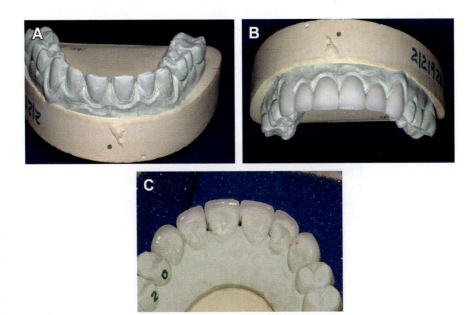

Fig. 7. (*A–C*) Veneers placed on model and checked for accuracy.

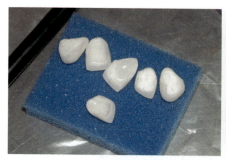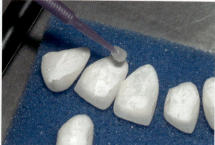

Fig. 8. Veneers silanated with Bis-Silane.

It is important for the practicing dentist to be knowledgeable in the diagnosis and treatment of dental fluorosis. Depending on the extent of fluorosis severity, several options exist to minimize unesthetic effects. For mild cases, a conservative approach, such as enamel microabrasion, can be performed; hydrochloric acid or finishing bur can be used for this purpose. Additionally, tooth bleaching or combination of both has been successful at minimizing superficial enamel opacities.[18–21] Composite resins are an option for moderate to severe cases, but may require knowledge of adhesive systems for optimum bonding strengths.[22,23] The finest and most durable restorative option for fluorotic teeth is the etched porcelain veneer restoration. For the patient discussed in this article, the use of bleaching followed by etched porcelain veneer restorations was used.

Tooth whitening has become an integral aspect of esthetic dentistry. Significant research efforts during the last decade have resulted in various innovative products and new application technologies. Cumulative data demonstrate that when used properly, peroxide-based tooth whiteners are safe and effective.[24–26]

Since its introduction more than two decades ago, the etched porcelain veneer restoration has proved to be a durable esthetic modality of treatment.[27,28] With the advent of high-strength porcelains, superior cements, and bonding agents, it is not unusual to provide a patient with maximum function and esthetics with minimal preparation using all-ceramic porcelain bonded restorations.

The dental professional should have knowledge of smile design and proper selection and use of restorative materials. Proper dentofacial evaluation and treatment planning is required for optimal esthetics. The incisal edge position of the maxillary central incisors relative to the upper lip should be established at the onset. This

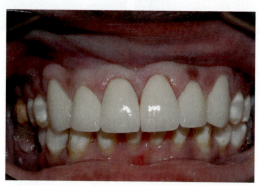

Fig. 9. Veneers cemented.

assessment is made with the patient's upper lip at rest using a millimeter ruler or a periodontal probe. The position of the maxillary central incisor can be either acceptable or unacceptable. An acceptable amount of incisal edge display at rest depends on the patient's age and sex. Establishment of the maxillary dental midline is determined relative to the facial midline.[29]

The golden proportion is used as a guideline to determine a pleasing esthetic appearance of the upper anterior teeth.[30,31] The golden proportion theory seems to be applicable to relate the successive widths of the maxillary anterior teeth if percentages are adjusted. A clinical examination was performed and the basic restorative work completed. The periodontal examination revealed the need for scaling and root planing to achieve gingival health. After scaling and root planing and healing phase were completed the patient's periodontal condition was re-evaluated. The result was a healthy periodontal status now ready for restorative dentistry.

The depth of the staining could not be determined. Teeth bleaching was introduced to reduce the discoloration and the necessity for more opaque veneers, thus creating a more natural appearance. However, it is generally not recommended that bonded restoration treatment be carried out immediately after bleaching treatment because the bleaching affects bond strength. The use of 10% sodium ascorbate gel (an antioxidant) can help the clinician to perform bonding procedures immediately after bleaching treatments.[32]

SUMMARY

This article discusses how to use a multistep process to conservatively achieve a successful esthetic result in a patient with severe dental fluorosis. Bleaching and porcelain veneers were used in this case to successfully address the needs of this patient. A combination of bleaching and porcelain veneer restoration can provide the patient maximum function and esthetics. Patient teeth have been treated with bleaching and/or microabrasion with some degree of success. However, predictable long-term results for stained discolored teeth can be achieved with resin bonded porcelain veneers (**Fig. 10**).

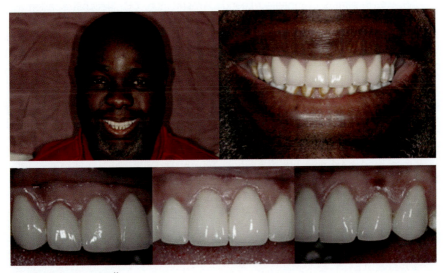

Fig. 10. One-year recall.

REFERENCES

1. Chu YM, Bergeron L, Chen YR. Bimaxillary protrusion: an overview of the surgical-orthodontic treatment. Semin Plast Surg 2009;23:32–9.
2. Bağlar S, Çolak H, Hamidi MM. Evaluation of novel microabrasion paste as a dental bleaching material and effects on enamel surface. J Esthet Restor Dent 2014. [Epub ahead of print].
3. Den Besten PK. Dental fluorosis: its use as a biomarker. Adv Dent Res 1994;8: 105–10.
4. Akosu TJ, Zoakah AI. Risk factors associated with dental fluorosis in Central Plateau State, Nigeria. Community Dent Oral Epidemiol 2008;36:144–8.
5. Yoder KM, Mabelya L, Robison VA, et al. Severe dental fluorosis in a Tanzanian population consuming water with negligible fluoride concentration. Community Dent Oral Epidemiol 1998;26:382–93.
6. Porcar C, Bronsoms J, Lopez-Bonet E, et al. Fluorosis, osteomalacia and pseudo-hyperparathyroidism in a patient with renal failure. Nephron 1998;79:234–5.
7. Dean HT, Arnold FA, Elvone E. Domestic water and dental caries. V. Additional studies of the relation of fluoride domestic waters to dental caries experience in 4425 white children aged 12 to 14 years of 13 cities in 4 states. Public Health Rep 1942;57:1155.
8. Rango T, Vengosh A, Jeuland M, et al. Fluoride exposure from groundwater as reflected by urinary fluoride and children's dental fluorosis in the Main Ethiopian Rift Valley. Sci Total Environ 2014;496:188–97.
9. Majumdar KK. Health impact of supplying safe drinking water containing fluoride below permissible level on fluorosis patients in a fluoride-endemic rural area of West Bengal. Indian J Public Health 2011;55:303–8.
10. Zhi C, Sun J. The quantitative epidemiologic study of endemic fluorosis. Chinese Journal of Control of Endemic Disease 1989;1:007.
11. Thylstrup A, Fejerskov O. Clinical appearance of dental fluorosis in permanent teeth in relation to histologic changes. Community Dent Oral Epidemiol 1978;6: 315–28.
12. Subcommittee on Health Effects of Ingested Fluoride (National Research Council). Health effects of ingested fluoride. Washington, DC: National Academy of Sciences; 1993.
13. Dean HT. Fluorine in the control of dental caries. J Am Dent Assoc 1956;52:1–8.
14. Dean HT. Endemic fluorosis and its relation to dental caries: 1938. Public Health Rep 2006;121(Suppl 1):213–9 [discussion: 212].
15. Harris NO, Garcia-Godoy F. Primary preventive dentistry. 5th edition. Stamford (CT): Appleton and Lange; 1999. p. 658.
16. de Castilho LS, e Ferreira EF, Perini E. Perceptions of adolescents and young people regarding endemic dental fluorosis in a rural area of Brazil: psychosocial suffering. Health Soc Care Community 2009;17(6):557–63.
17. Fantaye W, Anne A, Asgeir B, et al. Perception of dental fluorosis among adolescents living in urban areas of Ethiopia. Ethiop Med J 2003;41(1):35–44.
18. Riordan PJ. Perceptions of dental fluorosis. J Dent Res 1993;72(9):1268–74.
19. Pontes DG, Correa KM, Cohen-Carneiro F. Re-establishing esthetics of fluorosis-stained teeth using enamel microabrasion and dental bleaching techniques. Eur J Esthet Dent 2012;7:130–7.
20. Celik E, Tildiz G, Yazkan B. Comparison of enamel microabrasion with a combined approach to the esthetic management of fluorosed teeth. Oper Dent 2013;38(5):E134–43.

21. Loguercio AD, Correia LD, Zago C, et al. Clinical effectiveness of two microabrasion materials for the removal of enamel fluorosis stains. Oper Dent 2007;32: 531–8.
22. Knosel M, Attin R, Becker K, et al. A randomized CIE lab evaluation of external bleaching therapy effects on fluorotic enamel stains. Quintessence Int 2008;39: 391–9.
23. Ertuğrul F, Türkün M, Türkün LS, et al. Bond strength of different dentin bonding systems to fluorotic enamel. J Adhes Dent 2009;11(4):299–303.
24. Torres-Gallegos I, A Martinez-Castañon G, Loyola-Rodriguez JP, et al. Effectiveness of bonding resin-based composite to healthy and fluorotic enamel using total-etch and two self-etch adhesive systems. Dent Mater J 2012;31(6):1021–7.
25. Heymann HO, Swift EJ Jr, Bayne SC, et al. Clinical evaluation of two carbamide peroxide tooth-whitening agents. Compend Contin Educ Dent 1998;19(4): 359–62, 364–6, 369.
26. Li Y. Peroxide-containing tooth whiteners: an update on safety. Compend Contin Educ Dent 2000;21(Suppl 28):4–9.
27. Maggio B, Gallagher A, Bowman J, et al. Evaluation of a whitening gel designed to accelerate whitening. Compend Contin Educ Dent 2003;24(7):519–20, 523–6, 528,536.
28. Calamia JR. The current status of etched porcelain veneer restorations. J Indiana Dent Assoc 1993;72(5):10–5.
29. Calamia JR, Calamia CS. Porcelain laminate veneers: reasons for 25 years of success. Dent Clin North Am 2007;51(2):399–417, ix.
30. Spear FM, Kokich VG, Mathews DP. Interdisciplinary management of anterior dental esthetics. J Am Dent Assoc 2006;137(2):160–9.
31. Snow SR. Esthetic smile analysis of maxillary anterior tooth width: the golden percentage. J Esthet Dent 1999;11(4):177–84.
32. Garcia EJ, Mena-Serrano A, de Andrade AM, et al. Immediate bonding to bleached enamel treated with 10% sodium ascorbate gel: a case report with one-year follow-up. Eur J Esthet Dent 2012;7(2):154–62.

Comprehensive Risk-Based Diagnostically Driven Treatment Planning

Developing Sequentially Generated Treatment

Dean E. Kois, DMD, MSD, John C. Kois, DMD, MSD*

KEYWORDS

- Risk assessment • Full-mouth rehabilitation • Prognosis • Vertical dimension
- Kois deprogrammer • Biocorrosion • Esthetic • Adhesive

KEY POINTS

- Develop a systematic approach for comprehensive treatment planning.
- Focus on the 4 most important diagnostic categories: periodontal, biomechanical, functional, dentofacial.
- Develop and utilize critical risk parameters to minimize failure and maximize successful treatment strategies.
- Utilize minimally invasive strategies to minimize tooth reduction and future tooth sequelae.
- Use a sequential management strategy for large restorative cases so finances are not a barrier to executing necessary comprehensive care.

Dental health care is evolving by improving tooth mortality through advances in technology and preventative services. Unfortunately, dentists continue to primarily base treatment on a reparative model, in which therapy merely fixes the result of disease without addressing the cause of disease. The alternative or medical model is the term coined by psychiatrist R.D. Laing for the "set of procedures in which all doctors are trained."[1] The concept of disease is central to the medical model. In general, disease refers to some deviation from normal body functioning that has undesirable consequences for the affected individual. An important aspect of the medical model is that it regards disease signs (objective indicators such as an increased temperature) and symptoms (subjective feelings of distress expressed by the patient) as indicative of an underlying physical abnormality (pathology) within the individual. Understanding disease expression can be confusing due to inaccurately understanding science,

---

Disclosure: The authors have no financial interest.
Kois Center, LLC, 1001 Fairview Avenue North, Suite 2200, Seattle, WA 98109, USA
* Corresponding author.
E-mail address: info@koiscenter.com

Dent Clin N Am 59 (2015) 593–608
http://dx.doi.org/10.1016/j.cden.2015.03.001
0011-8532/15/$ – see front matter © 2015 Elsevier Inc. All rights reserved.

practitioner bias, or patient adaptation. According to the medical model, whenever possible medical treatment should be directed at the underlying pathology in an attempt to correct the abnormality and cure the disease. A comprehensive evaluation to determine the underlying cause of the disease will necessarily include chief concern, history, physical examination, ancillary tests if needed, diagnosis, treatment, and prognosis with and without treatment. "There can be several ways to treat a problem but there can only be one diagnosis".[2] When evaluating a fractured tooth, the reparative model would restore or fix the tooth without a definitive understanding of the underlying causes for the fracture. Did it fracture from an old restoration that structurally compromised the tooth, an unhealthy habit, tooth position, or some other reason or combination? The why must be both discovered and addressed to reduce the future risk and improve the prognosis of the diseased area or the tooth. For optimal outcomes this level of judgment may be more important than the operator's skill level.

The fundamental rationale for a comprehensive treatment approach is a long-term strategy for dental health commensurate with an enhanced level of wellness for patients. Dental care must therefore be directed through a comprehensive system that identifies health and disease as well as the potential risks to a patient undergoing treatment or refusing it. Risk to the dentition is identified by collecting objective data in an organized system. A diagnosis is formulated first and necessary treatment can be recommended thereafter. Treatment should always mitigate future risk and improve prognoses of the teeth and therefore decrease tooth mortality.

The following clinical example demonstrates a risk-based, diagnostically driven treatment planning approach by focusing on 4 key categories: periodontal, biomechanical, functional, dentofacial. In addition, our unique approach allowed the comprehensive clinical management of a patient with complex restorative needs. A full-mouth rehabilitation was completed sequentially without sacrificing the amount of dentistry necessary to restore health, comfort, function, and esthetics. The result exceeded the patient's expectation and was made financially possible by extending treatment over numerous years.

PATIENT BACKGROUND

The patient was a white male engineer in his late 40s (**Fig. 1**). His immediate chief concerns were the wear of his teeth, and the potholes on the biting surface of the posterior teeth. He stated that he could "see through the front teeth" (**Fig. 2**). The patient stated that the wear started many years ago but had been stable until recently, when he noticed that it had worsened. He has become increasingly more self-conscious about his smile, and reported that his "bite feels unstable and uneven". He also noted that he must consciously make an effort to find the "correct place" where his teeth fit together, and states that, "where my teeth fit together is not where my jaw feels most comfortable" (**Fig. 3**).

He was primarily concerned with functional longevity and future protection of his remaining teeth with esthetic improvement as a secondary benefit. He had been to several dental specialists seeking care and all had recommended a full-mouth reconstruction that would need to be done all at one time. The cost of this option had prevented him from proceeding with treatment. Using the diagnostically driven treatment planning approach, the full-mouth restoration could be completed sequentially, making it financially feasible.

MEDICAL HISTORY

The only remarkable finding in the medical history was a positive response to digestive disorders. The patient was diagnosed with gastroesophageal reflux disease (GERD) in

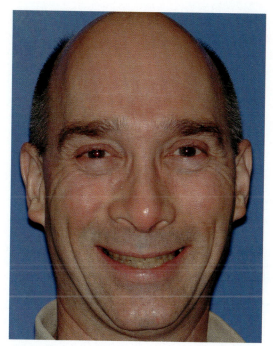

Fig. 1. Preoperative frontal full-face smile view.

1996 with an endoscopic procedure and, subsequently, proton pump inhibitor medication was used for 7 years. He reported no current medications except daily multivitamins.

DENTAL HISTORY

Overall, the patient reported favorable dental experiences. Minimal restorative care had been performed in the recent years. He had a nightguard fabricated 7 years previously in order to "protect his teeth from bruxism", but had not worn it.

Periodontal

The patient has maintained 6-month recare intervals for many years. He had isolated 4 mm probing depths in the maxillary and mandibular molars with little to no bleeding on probing and minimal attachment loss with no areas of site-specific bone loss

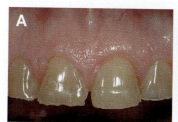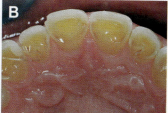

Fig. 2. (A) Preoperative retracted view of maxillary anterior teeth (facial). (B) Preoperative retracted view of maxillary anterior teeth (palatal).

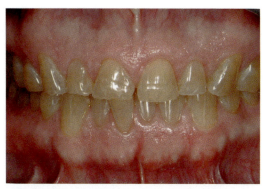

Fig. 3. Preoperative retracted maximum intercuspal position view.

(vertical defects) (**Fig. 4**). No increased genetic susceptibility was uncovered. There was no secondary occlusal traumatism. Mandibular tori and mandibular buccal exostoses were noted on teeth 19, 20, 29, and 30.

Biomechanical

All molars were structurally compromised with large multisurface alloy restorations present on teeth 2, 3, 14, 15, 30, and 31, and full coverage cast restorations on teeth 18 and 19 with an existing root canal therapy for tooth 19. The alloy restorations were over 30 years old with visible marginal discoloration. A caries risk assessment was performed and results were negative. No cavitations or defects were determined due to caries and he reported excessive soda consumption throughout the day. However, significant biocorrosion was evident on teeth 4–13, 20–22, and 27–29 (**Fig. 5**).

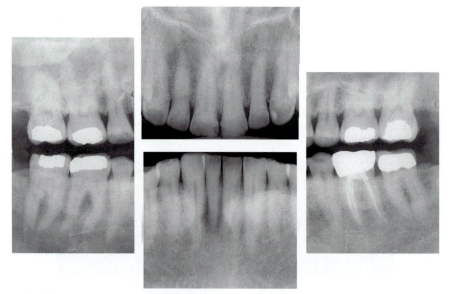

Fig. 4. Preoperative full-mouth radiographs.

A   B

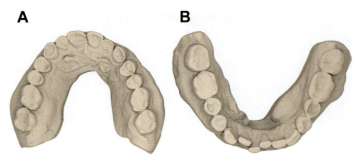

Fig. 5. Preoperative occlusal cast views (*A*) maxillary (*B*) mandibular.

The patient also reported tooth sensitivity on teeth 5, 8, and 20 and possible future pulpal pathology on teeth 2–5, 12–15, 30, and 31; significant loss of tooth structure from environmental damage was noted.

Functional

Severe attrition was noted on the anterior teeth (**Fig. 6**), although no primary occlusal traumatism could be detected. The patient reported pain in the muscles of mastication on the right side. Both the mandibular maximal opening (46 mm) and range of motion were within normal limits. During the assessment of the temporomandibular joint, no popping, clicking, or crepitus in the joints was noted. The immobilization test was positive on the right side and negative on the left side; the load test was negative bilaterally. No additional imaging of the joints was performed.

Dentofacial

The patient was unhappy with the color of his teeth. He considered them to be "too yellow" and wanted them whiter. His face height was normal with a slightly longer inferior third. A smile evaluation determined that the dental midlines were coincident. Tooth display was −4 mm in repose and 4 mm in high smile in the right cuspid region. The lip length was within normal limits at 22 mm. He showed medium lip dynamics in the maxillary arch with 8 mm of movement and medium lip dynamics with 5 mm of movement in the mandibular arch. The gingival architecture presented with horizontal

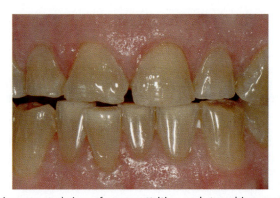

Fig. 6. Preoperative retracted view of severe attrition and stress biocorrosion.

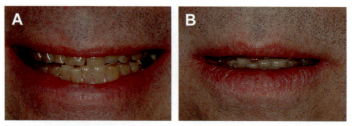

Fig. 7. (*A*) Preoperative frontal high smile view. (*B*) Preoperative lips in repose view.

symmetry and normal gingival scallop (**Fig. 7**).[3] The gingival scallop form was normal and mild crowding and rotations of the mandibular anterior teeth were present.

DIAGNOSIS

After comprehensive data collection, diagnoses were made in several specific categories. By compartmentalizing the data into the categories of periodontal, biomechanical, functional, and dentofacial, the clinician can use the data in an organized format to formulate the diagnoses for each category. The clinician must uncover any underlying diseases before specific tooth prognosis is determined and subsequent treatment is recommended or performed. Tooth prognosis is based on the likely course teeth will follow without treatment. Assigning prognosis to the remaining teeth is critical because treatment recommendations should always attempt to reduce risk and improve prognosis (**Fig. 8**). Careful consideration should always be made to not increase risk or worsen prognosis by providing treatment. When risk cannot be effectively reduced, our efforts are focused on improving prognosis by minimizing the contributing factors of disease that can be managed. For example, in a subtractive approach, circumferential tooth preparation for a structurally compromised tooth may further weaken the remaining tooth structure and increase the risk of irreversible pulpitis. If the reason for the tooth preparation was attrition, the compromise is even greater because the tooth is already shorter. In this situation, an additive approach would allow the practitioner the opportunity to return the tooth to a normal esthetic appearance, cover the unprotected dentin, and therefore, improve the prognosis biomechanically without increasing risk. This presents a problem because it would interfere with the occlusion.

Periodontal

AAP (American Academy of Periodontology)type II classification of periodontal disease. No other shared risk factors.

Risk profile: Low.

Prognosis: This patient has remained periodontally stable after scaling and root planing with continued recare intervals of 6 months. Therefore he received a good periodontal prognosis, without requiring more invasive periodontal therapy.

Biomechanical

Defective restorations (teeth 30 and 31); severe active biocorrosion (teeth 4–13, 20–22, and 27–29); structurally compromised teeth (teeth 2–5, 12–15, 19, 30, and 31).

Risk profile: High.

Prognosis: The dentition was compromised due to the number of structurally compromised teeth and the severe active biocorrosion of many of the remaining teeth.

Steve NAME **DIAGNOSTIC OPINION** AGE 48 DATE

RISK ASSESSMENT LOW *Acceptable* **MODERATE** *May require further attention* **HIGH** *Requires immediate attention*

PERIODONTAL
● LOW ○ MODERATE ○ HIGH Risk Assessment

- ☐ Gingivitis **(Gum)** (AAPI) Modified By:
- ■ Attachment Loss / Chronic Periodontitis **(Bone Loss)**
  - ● Mild (AAPII) ☐ Moderate (AAPIII) ☐ Severe (AAPIV)
    - ☐ Site Specific (Intrabony)
    - ☐ Horizontal Bone Loss
- ☐ Aggressive Periodontitis
- ☐ Secondary Occlusal Traumatism
- ☐ Abrasion
- ☐ Recession

- ☐ Posterior Bite Collapse
- ☐ Oral Pathology
- ☐ Impaction
- ☐ Missing Teeth
- ■ Other **Tori, exoxtosis**

PROGNOSIS Generalized *(Remaining Teeth)*
○ EXCELLENT ● GOOD ○ FAIR ○ POOR ○ HOPELESS
Specific *(Individual Teeth)*

BIOMECHANICAL
● LOW ○ MODERATE ○ HIGH Risk Assessment

- ☐ Caries
- ☐ Enamel Decalcification
- ☐ Defective Restorations
- ■ Questionable Restorations **30, 31**
- ☐ Xerostomia
- ■ Erosion **4–13, 20–22, 27–29**
- ■ Structural Compromises **2–5, 12–15, 19, 30, 31**
- ■ Pulpal Pathology **2–5, 12–15, 30, 31**

- ☐ Defective Root Canal Treatment Concerns
- ☐ Crown Margin Location Concerns
- ☐ Missing Teeth
- ☐ Other

PROGNOSIS Generalized *(Remaining Teeth)*
○ EXCELLENT ○ GOOD ○ FAIR ● POOR ○ HOPELESS
Specific *(Individual Teeth)*

FUNCTIONAL
○ LOW ● MODERATE ○ HIGH Risk Assessment

- ■ Attrition / Normal Force
  - ☐ Minimal ☐ Moderate ■ Severe
- ☐ Abnormal Attrition / Bruxism / Excessive Force
  - ☐ Minimal ☐ Moderate ☐ Severe
- ☐ Abfraction
- ☐ Primary Occlusal Traumatism
- ☐ TMD
- ☐ Abnormal Neuromuscular Habits
- ☐ Compromised Occlusal Vertical Dimension
- ■ Missing Teeth **1, 16, 17, 32**
- ☐ Other

- ☐ ACCEPTABLE FUNCTION
- ☐ CONSTRICTED CHEWING PATTERN
- ■ OCCLUSAL DYSFUNCTION (OSA, UARS)
- ☐ PARAFUNCTION (SLEEP BRUXISM)
- ☐ NEUROLOGIC DISORDERS

PROGNOSIS Generalized *(Remaining Teeth)*
○ EXCELLENT ○ GOOD ● FAIR ● POOR ○ HOPELESS
Specific *(Individual Teeth)*

DENTOFACIAL
○ LOW ● MODERATE ○ HIGH Risk Assessment

COLOR
- ☐ Developmental Disturbances ☐ Acceptable ■ Modify

FACIALLY RELATED TOOTH POSITION
1. Maxillary Incisal Edge Position ☐ Acceptable ■ Modify
2. Maxillary Posterior Occlusal Plane ☐ Acceptable ■ Modify
3. Mandibular Incisal Edge Position ☐ Acceptable ■ Modify
4. Mandibular Posterior Occlusal Plane ☐ Acceptable ■ Modify
5. Intra-arch Tooth Position *(Arrangement & Form)*
   - Midline ■ Acceptable ○ Modify
   - ☐ Left ☐ Right ☐ Axially Inclined
   - Crowding / Overlap **Lower Inc.** ☐ Acceptable ■ Modify
   - Diastema ■ Acceptable ○ Modify
   - Rotations ■ Acceptable ○ Modify

6a. Gingival Tissue Assessment MAXILLARY

Lip Dynamics	☐ Low	■ Medium	☐ High
	■ Acceptable		☐ Modify
Horizontal Symmetry	■ Acceptable		☐ Modify
Scallop / Form	☐ Flat	■ Normal	☐ High

6b. Gingival Tissue Assessment MANDIBULAR

Lip Dynamics	☐ Low	■ Medium	☐ High
	■ Acceptable		☐ Modify
Horizontal Symmetry	■ Acceptable		☐ Modify
Scallop / Form	☐ Flat	■ Normal	☐ High

- ☐ Missing Teeth
- ☐ Other

Patient's Vision *Function and Esthetics*
PROGNOSIS Generalized *(Remaining Teeth)*
○ EXCELLENT ○ GOOD ○ FAIR ● POOR ○ HOPELESS
Specific *(Individual Teeth)*

v 2012.2 © Kois Center, LLC

To reorder, please visit: **www.koiscenter.com**

Fig. 8. The diagnostic opinion form, Kois Center, LLC. (*Courtesy of* Kois Center, LLC, Seattle, WA; with permission.)

The structurally compromised teeth continue to be at risk for fracture and the biocorrosion has resulted in teeth with minimal enamel and even more vulnerable exposed dentin.[4] The teeth are therefore more susceptible to additional environmental damage from acidic foods and beverages, abrasive foods, and dentrifices. This patient was given a poor biomechanical prognosis.

Functional

Severe attrition; missing teeth (1, 16, 17, and 32); occlusal dysfunction.

Risk profile: Moderate.

Prognosis: The occlusal instability and attrition was determined to be multifactorial. Tooth position, years of attrition, tooth structure loss and unfavorable load (patient admitted to squeezing to make the teeth fit together) on the teeth have contributed to the progressive current state of the occlusion. The negative sequelae of this multifactorial problem seemed to have been consistent for many years. However, the patient reported that "things have gotten worse more recently", indicating active tooth structure loss. The teeth will likely lose more tooth structure at an unknown rate due to his diet and shared risk factors, further exacerbating his occlusal disease. Therefore, this patient was given a fair to poor functional prognosis.

Dentofacial

Discolored teeth; mild crowding; inadequate tooth display.

Risk profile: Moderate.

Prognosis: The amount of tooth structure lost from dental biocorrosion and attrition have resulted in the teeth appearing too short in the face. The yellow color bothers the patient. Tooth display is below average. Vital tooth bleaching would be unsuccessful in a patient with this much enamel loss. Color and tooth display are not correctable without restorative intervention. This patient was assigned a poor dentofacial prognosis.

Medical Precautions

American Society of Anesthesiologists Physical Classification 1 (ASA1) gastritis/concern for GERD.

Risk profile: Low.

Prognosis: Monitoring the patient for GERD should be a sufficient management strategy. This patient was given a good medical prognosis.

TREATMENT

A sequential full-mouth rehabilitation in a mutually protected, musculoskeletally stable position, focusing on the patient's goals was carried out through composite onlays initially and ultimately with the placement of adhesively retained reinforced ceramic indirect restorations and cohesively retained restorations. The restorative treatment was designed to protect the teeth from further structure loss and restore a harmonious balanced occlusion.

TREATMENT SEQUENCE

The existing maximum intercuspal position (tooth-based) exhibited dysfunction and was determined to not be reliable due to the tooth structure loss and active functional concerns previously discussed in the data collection. Centric relation (joint-based) was used as the reference position of the mandible to establish an orthopedically stable position and ensure that symptoms would be eliminated (surrogate end point). To identify the position of centric relation, a Kois Deprogrammer (Kois Center LLC., Seattle, WA) was used (**Fig. 9**) to test or preview the occlusal outcome. To accomplish this, the deprogrammer was designed and inserted with 1.0–1.5 mm of occlusal space in the second molar region. This allowed the patient to deprogram by not allowing any tooth-guided occlusion, which tests the patient's ability to retrain their brain and develop a new neural pathway of the muscles to seat the condyles.[5] All

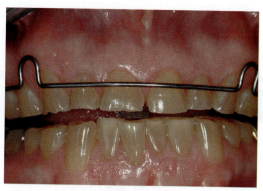

Fig. 9. Frontal view of the Kois Deprogrammer in place.

temporomandibular symptoms resolved after wearing the deprogrammer for 1 week. The Kois Dentofacial Analyzer (Panadent, Colton, CA) was used to communicate essential functional (arithmetical relationship to the rotational axis) and esthetic (symmetry of the maxillary arch to the face) parameters for the maxillary diagnostic cast transfer to the Panadent articulator (Magnetic Model PCH Articulator, Panadent, Colton, CA).[6]

The Kois Dentofacial Analyzer transfers the way the teeth actually appear in the face in contrast to other facebows that transfer the casts based purely on functional relationships, which incorporate errors in the esthetic relationship of the occlusal plane. This is accomplished by first aligning the vertical rod with the facial midline not the dental midline, which adds a valuable communication key for treatment planning and laboratory communication. The bow is then seated against only the most inferior tooth in the maxillary arch and then horizontally aligned level left to right and front to back; not just seated against the teeth (**Fig. 10**A). In this way, the position of the maxillary teeth relative to the face will be easier to evaluate. The vertical wall on the index tray is positioned against the facial surface of the maxillary central incisors to relate the position of the maxillary cast functionally to an arithmetically predetermined rotational

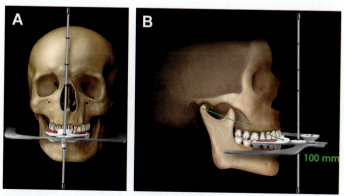

Fig. 10. (*A*) Kois Dentofacial Analyzer frontal view, skeletal representation. (*B*) Kois Dentofacial Analyzer lateral view, skeletal representation.

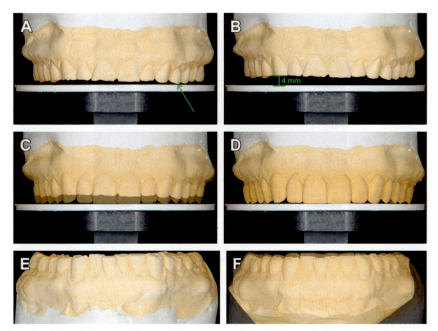

Fig. 11. (*A*) Frontal view of the maxillary diagnostic cast mounted with the Kois Dentofacial Analyzer in the esthetic plane. Note tooth 12 is touching the platform and vertically is the longest tooth in the esthetic plane. (*B*) The mounting platform is lowered to accommodate the increased tooth length. (*C*) Diagnostic waxing of the entire maxillary arch with increased tooth length. (*D*) Duplicated cast of the maxillary diagnostic wax-up demonstrating horizontal symmetry to the esthetic plane. (*E*) Frontal view of the mandibular diagnostic cast. (*F*) Diagnostic waxing of the entire mandibular arch with increased tooth length.

axis of 100 mm (see **Fig. 10**B). The mandibular diagnostic cast was then mounted with the centric relation record obtained using the Kois Deprogrammer.

After the diagnostic mounting, the mounting platform can be used to develop the critical esthetic modifications. Tooth 12 was the longest tooth in the face and is the only tooth that touches the platform (**Fig. 11**A). The platform, however, now represents what would appear horizontal in the face but does not determine the tooth length

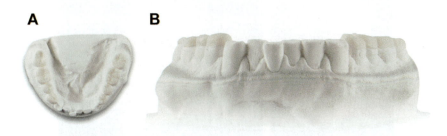

Fig. 12. (*A*) Mandibular cast occlusal view of the no-preparation composite onlays. (*B*) Mandibular cast frontal view of the no-preparation composite onlays.

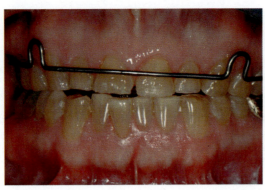

Fig. 13. Retracted view of the Kois Deprogrammer in place and mandibular no-preparation onlays seated.

needed to optimize facial esthetics. This decision is determined by the dentofacial risk analysis done previously.

Maxillary and mandibular tooth length was determined to be deficient. The decision to lengthen the maxillary arch was first determined by the deficiency of the right cuspid display in repose.[7] This determination required an additional 4 mm of tooth length to the right maxillary cuspid and then the mounting platform was lowered to accommodate this additional tooth length (see **Fig. 11**B). Now the platform can also provide necessary guidelines for treatment planning and the diagnostic wax-up because it represents what is level in the face (see **Fig. 11**C). The diagnostic wax-up or definitive restorations can now be completed with the assurance of dentofacial harmony (see **Fig. 11**D).

In this way, the Panadent system is the only semi-adjustable articulator that allows adding length to the maxillary arch without disrupting the esthetics of the maxillary occlusal plane. In other semi-adjustable articulators, when length is added to the maxillary arch, the incisal pin length is increased, which adversely affects the cant of the anterior-posterior occlusal plane. In contrast, length was added by moving the platform inferiorly to add the maxillary tooth length without changing the incisal

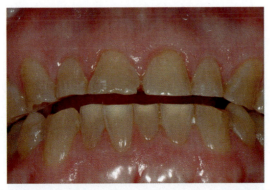

Fig. 14. Retracted maximum intercuspal view of the anterior relationship before anterior tooth preparation.

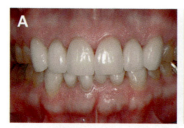
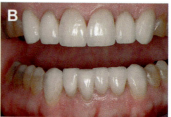

Fig. 15. (*A*) Postoperative retracted maximum intercuspal position view of anterior restorations. (*B*) Postoperative retracted slight opening to demonstrate transitional posterior restorations with definitive anterior restorations.

pin so the esthetic plane orientation is not altered in the face. This facebow system uses the esthetic plane, which is the correct plane to use for smile design, because it is the plane that is visible when the patient smiles. The mandibular arch was then waxed to accommodate the change in the maxillary arch and the face, which substantially further increased the occlusal vertical dimension (OVD) (see **Fig. 11**E, F).[8] The diagnostic wax-up was created at the centric relation transferred previously from the Kois Deprogrammer.

No-preparation occlusal onlays were fabricated from the wax-up with resin composite (Radica, Dentsply Ceramco, York, PA) (**Fig. 12**). Clinically, with the Kois Deprogrammer in place to control OVD in centric relation, the no-preparation resin composite onlays were bonded individually on teeth 18–21 and 28–31 and seated with resin composite (SonicFill, Kerr, Orange, CA) (**Fig. 13**). The occlusion was refined to achieve equal bilateral simultaneous contact using the same Kois Deprogrammer, which facilitates the adjustment. Next, at the same appointment, teeth 6–11 and 22–27 were prepared for anterior adhesively retained all-ceramic restorations. Minimally invasive protocols were used for tooth preparations because an additive strategy was being used and the OVD was increased, which provided additional occlusal clearance for the restorative materials (**Fig. 14**).

The definitive restorations for teeth 6–11 and 22–27 were seated at the subsequent appointment. After the provisionals were removed, a tooth cleansing protocol with an airborne particle abrasion unit was performed using 40 psi, 27 μm aluminous oxide with a 0.381 mm (0.015 inch) tip (Prep Start H$_2$O, Danville Materials, San Ramon,

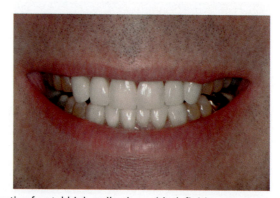

Fig. 16. Postoperative frontal high smile view with definitive anterior restorations.

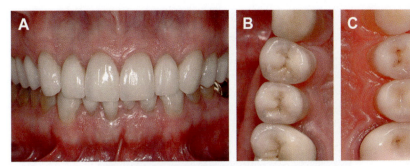

Fig. 17. (*A*) Postoperative retracted maximum intercuspal position view with entire maxilla restored. (*B*) Postoperative occlusal view of the maxillary posterior right side. (*C*) Postoperative occlusal view of the maxillary posterior left side.

CA).[9] Teeth 6–11 were restored with reinforced lithium disilicate restorations (IPS e.max, Ivoclar Vivadent, Amherst, NY) to improve esthetics, cover exposed areas of dentin and manage the anterior determinants of occlusion. Teeth 22–27 were restored with reinforced lithium disilicate veneers (IPS e.max, Ivoclar Vivadent, Amherst, NY) and all were adhesively luted[10] (RelyX Veneer, 3M ESPE, St Paul, MN). The adhesive bonding protocol was used to manage the tooth and material substrates to maximize bond strength and longevity. Cuspid rise was used as the occlusal scheme to control lateral interferences of the posterior teeth but meticulous management of the envelope of function was directed to minimize friction and load on the anterior teeth (**Figs. 15** and **16**).

Over the next 4 years, the posterior segments were definitively restored. First, the maxillary posterior teeth were completed (**Fig. 17**) by quadrant, using a combination of adhesively retained bonded onlays (teeth 4, 5, 12, and 13) (IPS e.max, Ivoclar Vivadent, Amherst, NY) and cohesively retained crowns (teeth 2, 3, 14, and 15) (**Fig. 18**).

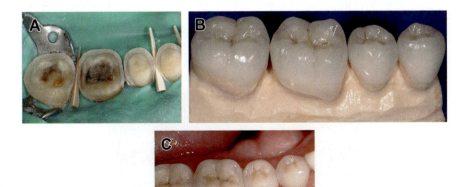

Fig. 18. (*A*) Tooth preparations of the mandibular posterior right side. (*B*) Laboratory image of the mandibular posterior right reinforced lithium disilicate restorations. (*C*) Postoperative occlusal view of the mandibular posterior right side.

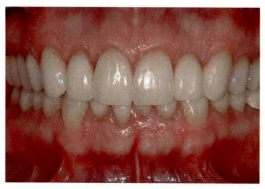

Fig. 19. Postoperative retracted maximum intercuspal position view.

This allowed the maxillary occlusal plane to be optimized before finalizing the mandibular restorations. In the next phase, quadrant dentistry could be facilitated to transition the temporary composite overlays to indirect restorations. Tooth 18 had irreversible pulpitis that required root canal therapy and (teeth 18 and 19) were restored with metal ceramic crowns to take advantage of a circumferential bevel.[11] Adhesively retained bonded onlays (teeth 20, 21, and 28–31) (IPS e.max, Ivoclar Vivadent, Amherst, NY) were used for the remaining mandibular teeth.

DISCUSSION

Because of the biomechanical concerns of active biocorrosion and active frictional loss of tooth structure from dysfunction, an additive strategy was used for treatment. In addition, many of the posterior teeth had very little enamel, at least 2 mm of tooth structure was already lost. Preparing those teeth with an additional 2 mm would certainly have added risk for pulpal pathology and eliminated the critical enamel ring necessary for successful bonding protocols.[12] The preparation design on worn teeth does not provide the same anatomic occlusal configuration of enamel and dentin to provide optimal adhesive bonding. The amount of remaining enamel in posterior teeth is proportional to the amount of tooth reduction necessary for the preparation.

The dentofacial determinants also indicated additional tooth length would be esthetically more pleasing. This would also reduce the esthetic risk. Therefore, the

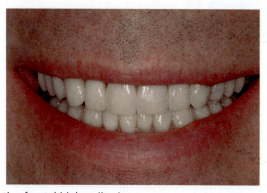

Fig. 20. Postoperative frontal high smile view.

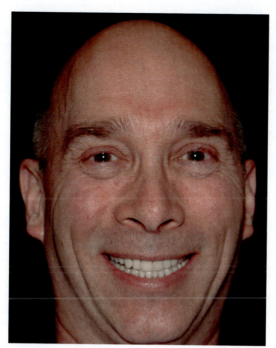

Fig. 21. Postoperative frontal full-face smile view.

thorough pretreatment diagnoses provided an understanding that the OVD could be opened for this patient, resulting in the need for only minimal tooth reduction.

Sequential management of this full-mouth reconstruction was initiated as a result of the financial constraints of the patient. This strategy gives more patients who need comprehensive care an opportunity to receive care. The no-preparation composite overlays have no structural impact on the teeth (ie, they do not increase risk), and they also facilitated management of the occlusion for sequential restoration placement.

COMMENTARY

The final result exceeded the patient's expectations. By identifying the patient's individual risk factors, periodontally, biomechanically, functionally, and dentofacially, a

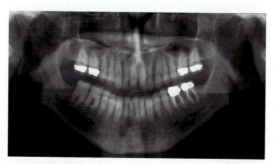

Fig. 22. Postoperative panograph.

treatment plan was designed and executed to minimize additional risk to the remaining dentition. Unfortunately, when the most appropriate treatment requires an increase in the patient's OVD, many patients cannot afford to undergo the treatment even though it would reduce their risk. However, this particular type of sequential phasing maintains the patient's specific goals for treatment and provides the clinician with an opportunity to offer the necessary care without unnecessary compromises (**Figs. 19–22**).

ACKNOWLEDGMENTS

Ceramics by Steve McGowan, Arcus Laboratory, Bothell, WA.

Composite Overlays by Claudio Bucceri, Swiss Dental & Technical Art.

REFERENCES

1. Laing R. The politics of the family and other essays. New York: Pantheon Books; 1971.
2. Amsterdam M. Periodontal prosthesis: twenty-five years in retrospect. Part V. Final treatment plan. Compend Contin Educ Dent 1984;5(7):577–89.
3. Tjan AH, Miller GD, The JG. Some esthetic factors in a smile. J Prosthet Dent 1984;51(1):24–8.
4. Grippo JO, Chaiyabutr Y, Kois JC. Effects of cyclic fatigue stress-biocorrosion on noncarious cervical lesions. J Esthet Restor Dent 2013;25(4):265–72.
5. Graybiel AM. How the brain makes and breaks habits. Sci Am 2014;310(6): 39–43.
6. Kois JC, Kois DE, Chaiyabutr Y. Occlusal errors generated at the maxillary incisal edge position related to discrepancies in the arbitrary horizontal axis location and to the thickness of the interocclusal record. J Prosthet Dent 2013;110(5):414–9.
7. Misch CE. Guidelines for maxillary incisal edge position-a pilot study: the key is the canine. J Prosthodont 2008;17(2):130–4.
8. Kois JC, Phillips KM. Occlusal vertical dimension: alteration concerns. Compend Contin Educ Dent 1997;18(12):1169–74.
9. Chaiyabutr Y, Kois JC. The effect of tooth-preparation cleansing protocol on the bond strength of self-adhesive resin cement to dentin contaminated with a hemostatic agent. Oper Dent 2011;36(1):18–26.
10. Chaiyabutr Y, Kois JC. The effects of tooth preparation cleansing protocols on the bond strength of self-adhesive resin luting cement to contaminated dentin. Oper Dent 2008;33(5):556–63.
11. Barkhordar RA, Radke R, Abbasi J. Effect of metal collars on resistance of endodontically treated teeth to root fracture. J Prosthet Dent 1989;61(6):676–8.
12. Kois DE, Chiabutyr Y, Kois JC. Comparison of load fatigue performance of posterior ceramic onlays restorations under different preparation designs. Compend Contin Educ Dent 2012;33(Spec No 2):2–9.

Full Mouth Rehabilitation Determined by Anterior Tooth Position

Nicholas J. Giannuzzi, DDS[a],*, Shawn Davaie Motlagh, DDS[b]

KEYWORDS

- Smile evaluation • Incisal edge position • Diagnostic wax-up

KEY POINTS

- When patients seek cosmetic dentistry, their main concern is how their new smile is going to appear.
- In trying to achieve a patient's desire for a more beautiful smile, a careful and comprehensive analysis must be completed to insure the desired outcome is achievable and will function for many years to come.
- The clinician's primary goal is to restore the patient's dentition to ideal form and function. Starting with the smile design process, the ideal upper central incisal edge position should be determined relative to maxillary lip.
- Once the ideal upper central incisal edge position is found, the remaining anterior teeth can be positioned and become the determinates for the posterior restorations.
- The posterior teeth and occlusion can be worked out to establish immediate posterior disclusion in lateral excursions.
- The restorations placed will provide years of service as long as function is incorporated into their design.
- Full mouth rehabilitations need to be done in a systematic way to ensure all the parameters of an esthetic and functional outcome are achieved.

PATIENT BACKGROUND

A 48-year-old female patient presented to the New York University College of Dentistry Honors Esthetics clinic for an evaluation.[1–3] Her chief complaint was a desire for a more beautiful smile.

MEDICAL HISTORY

The medical history contained no significant findings.

The authors have nothing to disclose.
[a] NYU Honors Program in Aesthetics, Department of Cariology and Comprehensive Care, New York City, 345 E 24th street, NY 10010, USA; [b] Private Practice, 10 Norton street, Irvine, CA 92612, USA
* Corresponding author.
E-mail address: njgdds@optonline.net

DENTAL HISTORY

The dental history contained mild plaque buildup, no calculus, and no visible peri-odontal disease. Periodontal pocketing was within normal limits with slight inflamma-tion. No visible caries. Generalized attrition was present due to bruxism.

SMILE EVALUATION (SEE INITIAL FORM)

It was noted that the patient had severe wear, combined with incisal edge chipping, in addition to an uneven smile line (**Figs. 1–3**). The anterior teeth were too square and not in an ideal width-to-length proportion. The posterior teeth were worn, and canine guid-ance needed to be re-established. The gingival zeniths of the central incisors were not in an ideal position. The patient has a low lip line that is not reveal these gingival zenith discrepancies, so the goal of treatment was to try to make the gingival zeniths more favorable without the need for osseous crown lengthening. Even though the gingival zeniths did not show, it was necessary to alter them as much as possible to help the technician create a proper emergence profile and contour in the final restorations. Material selection would be critical in this case. Strength as well as esthetics was necessary. Material choices included full gold, porcelain fused to metal, zirconium, or lithium disilicate. The patient expressed a desire for esthetic restorations. E-Max lithium disilicate (Ivoclar/Vivadent, Amherst, NY, USA) restorations were chosen because of their strength and esthetic properties. To establish the goals, the authors outlined that a full mouth rehabilitation was necessary with a systematic approach.

DIAGNOSTIC AIDS
Study Casts

Two sets of diagnostic casts were obtained. One set was used to establish the treat-ment plan and to have a record of the patient's original condition. The second set was sent to the laboratory with instructions for the diagnostic wax-up. The prescription to the laboratory must be detailed. The midline, upper central incisor desired length and width, and any gingival recontouring need to be conveyed to the laboratory technician.

DIAGNOSTIC WAX-UP

When performing a full mouth rehabilitation, it is imperative to establish where the anterior teeth need to be first and then restore the posterior teeth to allow function. Anterior guidance with posterior disclusion in lateral excursions will prevent the resto-rations from failing prematurely. Using smile design principles, it is necessary to deter-mine where the incisal edge of the central incisors should be located. This determination can be done in the mouth with a composite mockup, digitally using photos and a calibrated ruler, or by measuring directly on the patient. Once the incisal edge position is determined, the ideal width-to-length ratio of the central incisor (approximately 80%) can be ascertained. Using the principles of the Golden Propor-tion, the rest of the anterior teeth can be waxed. Study models (**Figs. 4–6**) of the pa-tient with a centric relation (CR) bite,[4] using bimanual manipulation, was sent to the laboratory. The prescription to the laboratory indicated the need to lengthen the cen-tral incisors by 3 mm. The vertical dimension would need to be opened posteriorly approximately 1 mm to achieve this. The diagnostic wax-up (**Figs. 7–9**) serves as a template to re-establish the patient's occlusion and anterior teeth. Ideal forms are established in wax and can be altered and adjusted in the patient's mouth.

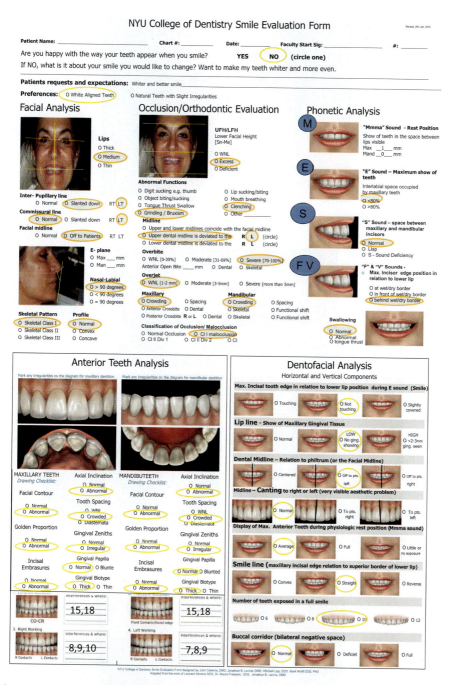

Fig. 1. NYU smile evaluation form. (*Courtesy of* John Calamia, DMD; Mitchell Lipp, DDS; and Jonathan B. Levine, DMD, GoSMILE Aesthetics, 923 5th Avenue, New York, NY 10021; *Adapted from* Leonard Abrams, 255 South Seventeenth Street, Philadelphia, PA 19103, 1987; and Dr Mauro Fradeani, Esthetic Rehabilitation in Fixed Prosthodontics Quintessence Publishing Co, Inc, Carol Stream, IL, 2004.)

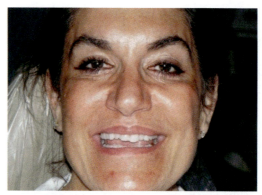

Fig. 2. Full face preoperatively.

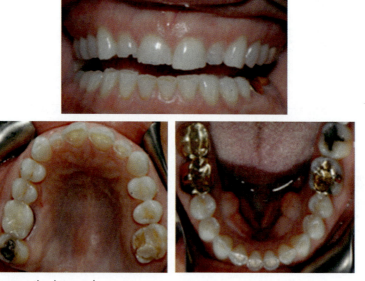

Fig. 3. Preoperative intraoral.

Diagnostic Models

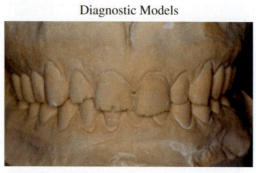

Fig. 4. Study model showing uneven and chipped and teeth.

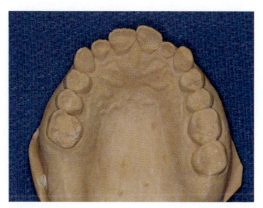

Fig. 5. Occlusal view showing wear.

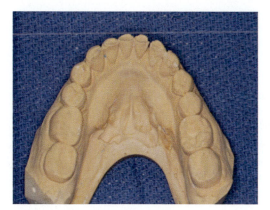

Fig. 6. Lower model showing wear.

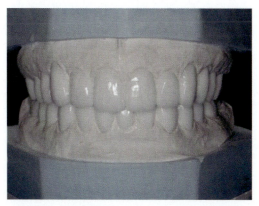

Fig. 7. Diagnostic wax-up at new VDO.

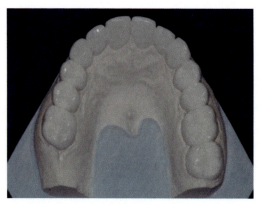

Fig. 8. Wax-up showing full contours and better arch form.

PATIENT'S PROBLEMS LIST

1. Generalized wear
2. Uneven smile line
3. Uneven gingival zeniths
4. Loss of vertical dimension of occlusion (VDO)

DIAGNOSIS

The diagnosis was generalized wear with loss of VDO.

TREATMENT PLAN

- Re-establish VDO and establish canine guidance with Emax pressed crowns teeth numbers 3–15, 18–21, 28–31, and
- Emax pressed veneers numbers 22–27

RISKS

Because of the patient's past history, ceramic breakage is a risk. Building a protected canine-guided occlusion will help reduce this risk by eliminating interferences that could cause fractures. The patient needs to be aware that regular re-care visits are

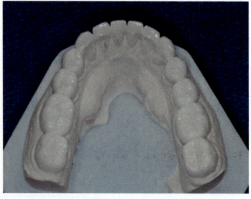

Fig. 9. Lower wax-up with restored contours.

necessary to help maintain the restorations. The patient was also given a night guard to help prevent nocturnal bruxism.

PROGNOSIS

The prognosis was excellent to good: before restoring this case, the patient was informed of what was expected of her to maintain the restorations. Diligent home care as well as regular recalls was necessary. The restorations could be compromised if the patient stopped being involved with their care.

TREATMENT SEQUENCE

Full mouth rehabilitation sequence
1. Diagnostic records
2. Mounted CR study models
3. Diagnostic wax-up

Stage 1
- Prepare maxillary arch and fabricate provisional (establish upper incisal edge position)

Stage 2
- Prepare mandibular arch and fabricate provisional

Stage 3
- Monitor patient and make any necessary adjustments (cosmetic or functional)

Stage 4
- Restore posterior teeth using anterior provisionals at established VDO

Stage 5
- Restore anterior teeth

Stage 1: Preparation and Provisionals

Upper and lower arches were prepared and a provisional (**Figs. 10** and **11**) was fabricated at individual appointments. A gingivectomy of teeth numbers 8 and 9 was performed using a diode laser. The gingival zeniths of numbers 8 and 9 were altered to maintain biologic width. The gingival zeniths were slightly more incisal than ideal but because of the patient's low lip line this was not an esthetic concern. Osseous surgery was avoided and the patient was happy with the result of the altered gingival levels.

The provisional restorations were made from Luxatemp (DMG America, Englewood, NJ, USA) using a putty matrix fabricated from the diagnostic wax-up. The occlusion was equilibrated to establish CR = CO and to establish canine guidance.[5] These provisionals acted as a guide for the final restorations. The patient wore the provisionals for 3 months to ensure she was comfortable with the new VDO.

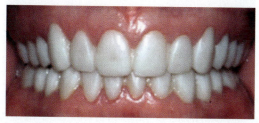

Fig. 10. Retracted view of provisionals at 3 months (note the periodontal health).

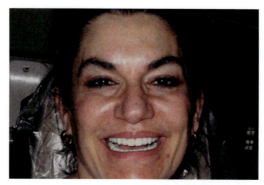

Fig. 11. Full face smile of provisional showing rejuvenated smile.

FINAL RESTORATIONS
Posterior Teeth

The patient was comfortable at her new VDO. At no time during the 3-month provisional stage did the patient feel discomfort or fracture any restorations. It was necessary to keep this VDO and established canine guidance in the final restorations. To achieve this goal, it was necessary to control the case by restoring the posterior teeth first. This restoration was accomplished by sectioning the provisional distal to canines (**Figs. 12** and **13**). The anterior provisionals held the current vertical and were verified using a caliper (**Fig. 14**). With the anterior portion of the provisional restoration in place, the laboratory technician was able to design the posterior occlusal tables and incorporate immediate disclusion during excursive movements (canine guidance) (**Figs. 15–18**).

E-Max crowns were made for teeth numbers 3, 4, 5, 12, 13, 14, 15.

The posterior restorations were cemented with a resin cement (RelyX Unicem (3M ESPE, St. Paul, MN, USA)) and were equilibrated to ensure CR = CO, and no interferences were present.

Anterior Teeth

The anterior teeth could now be restored because an established and stable posterior occlusion at the correct VDO had been created. E-Max Crowns were made for teeth numbers 6 to 11, and E-Max veneers were made for teeth numbers 22 to 27. The stump shade (**Fig. 19**) was taken to allow the laboratory technician to match the veneers and crowns because of the thickness variation of the different restorations. The laboratory was also sent a stick bite to show the facial midline and horizontal plane (**Fig. 20**).

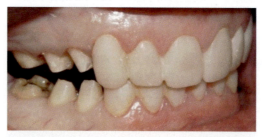

Fig. 12. Right lateral view with posterior provisionals removed at new VDO held by anterior provisionals.

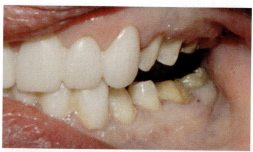

Fig. 13. Left lateral view with posterior provisionals removed at new VDO held by anterior provisionals.

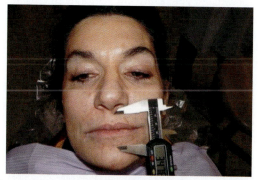

Fig. 14. Digital caliper used to ensure VDO established is maintained when fabricating final restorations.

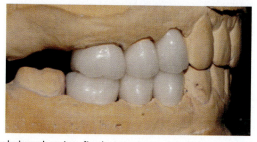

Fig. 15. Right lateral view showing final posterior restorations at new VDO.

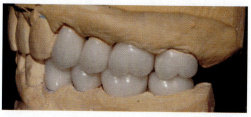

Fig. 16. Left lateral view showing final posterior restorations at new VDO.

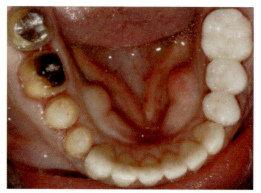

Fig. 17. Lower occlusal with left side permanent. Restorations cemented.

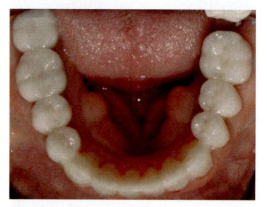

Fig. 18. Final lower posterior restorations seated.

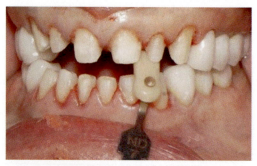

Fig. 19. Stump shade being established.

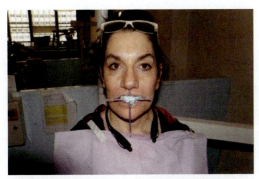

Fig. 20. Final bite registration with bite sticks to establish midline and occlusal plane.

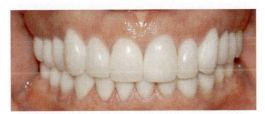

Fig. 21. Anterior retracted view, final restorations.

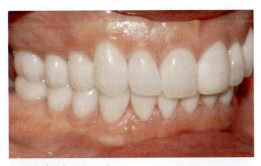

Fig. 22. Right lateral view, final restorations.

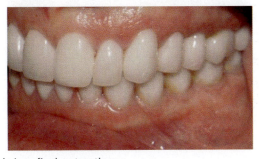

Fig. 23. Left lateral view, final restorations.

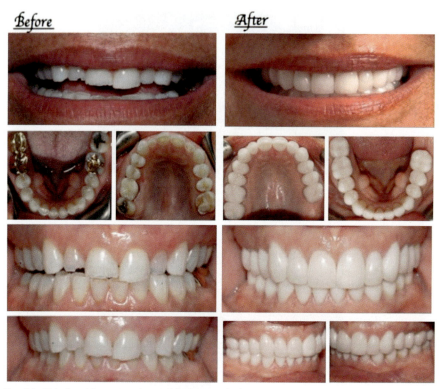

Fig. 24. Side-by-side comparison of before and after.

The upper anterior crowns were cemented with RelyX Unicem, and the lower veneers were bonded with a total etch technique using Prime & Bond NT (Dentsply, York, PA, USA) and Choice 2 (Bisco, Schaumburg, IL, USA) resin cement. Final equilibration was completed and a night guard was fabricated for the patient to wear. Final results are shown in **Figs. 21–26**.

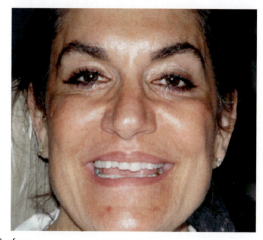

Fig. 25. Full face before.

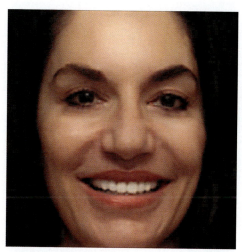

Fig. 26. Full face after with rejuvenated smile.

SUMMARY

A systematic approach was used to re-establish the patient's occlusion as well as to achieve the esthetic desires of the patient. Treatment planning is the cornerstone for any esthetic case. Having a predetermined plan will enable the clinician to systematically restore a dentition to ideal form and function. One must always have esthetics in mind while restoring complex cases. Establishing the position of the anterior teeth first enables the clinician to achieve the optimum esthetic result. Esthetics is of foremost importance, but function is paramount to the longevity and success of the restorations. Proper posterior support and canine guidance are necessary to ensure the restorations will remain functional for many years to come.

REFERENCES

1. Spear FM, Kokich VG, Mathews DP. Interdisciplinary management of anterior dental esthetics. J Am Dent Assoc 2006;137:160–9.
2. Morley J, Eubank J. Macroesthetic elements of smile design. J Am Dent Assoc 2001;132:39–45.
3. McLaren E, Phong TC. Smile analysis and esthetic design: in the zone. Inside Dent 2009;5:44–8.
4. Dawson P. Determining centric relation. In: Dolan J, Nebel J, editors. Functional occlusion: from TMJ to smile design. St. Louis (MO): Mosby, Inc; 2007. p. 75–83.
5. Spear FM. Occlusion in the new millennium: the controversy continues. Signature 2001;7:18–21.

Proportional Smile Design

Using the Recurring Esthetic Dental Proportion to Correlate the Widths and Lengths of the Maxillary Anterior Teeth with the Size of the Face

Daniel H. Ward, DDS, FAGD, FACD, FICD[a,b]

KEYWORDS

- Proportional smile design • RED proportion • Central incisor width/length ratio
- Tooth/face proportion

KEY POINTS

- Proportional smile design can be used to design a smile in harmony with the face. A smile created with the 78% width/length ratio of the maxillary central incisor has been shown to be preferred by dentists surveyed.
- Keeping the relative lengths of the teeth consistent with the height of the patient is recommended.
- A method of determining the relative widths of the maxillary anterior teeth should be used.
- Producing an imaged view of the recommended smile before active treatment is important to allow discussion and input from the patient to achieve pleasing results.

INTRODUCTION

Dentists and laboratory technicians have an important role in creating pleasing smiles for their patients. Methods that can predictably satisfy the patient should be used. Studies have measured the sizes and key proportions of the natural teeth.[1,2] Most people have variations in their smile that deviate from the published standards for ideal smiles. Orthodontic treatment is performed on a significant population of patients who are not satisfied with what nature has given them in their smiles. People spend significant amounts of money with plastic surgeons and dermatologists to look different than what was their natural appearance. Do we as dentists always want to give patients a smile that mirrors what is often found in nature, such as crowded, overlapped, and twisted teeth, malocclusions or diastemas (**Figs. 1** and **2**)? Do we want to

The author has nothing to disclose.
[a] Section of Restorative and Prosthetic Dentistry, The Ohio State University, College of Dentistry, 305 W Twelfth Ave Columbus, OH 43210, USA; [b] Private Practice, 1080 Polaris Parkway, Suite130, Columbus, OH 43240, USA
E-mail address: dward@columbus.rr.com

dental.theclinics.com

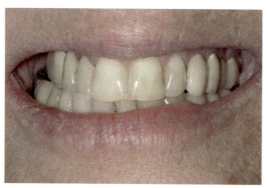

Fig. 1. Crowded teeth with malocclusion.

design smiles so they mimic the sizes and proportions found in nature? Should the use of proportions that are preferred by dentists be considered in addition to the proportions observed in nature?

THE GOLDEN PROPORTION

The golden proportion has been considered the standard by many for determining the ideal widths of the anterior teeth.[3,4] Based on formulas defined by ancient Greek mathematicians, the proportion has developed mythical connotations (**Fig. 3**).[5] Although often cited as the reference for designing smiles it has been this author's observance that smiles supposedly designed by this method were not conformant with this practice. When the proportions of natural anterior teeth were evaluated in numerous studies, the golden proportion was not found to be the predominant proportion observed.[6,7]

NATURAL PROPORTIONS

Studies have been conducted worldwide to determine the proportions of the teeth. Results vary according to location. Preston[8] observed that the average frontal tooth to tooth width proportion of North American dental students was 66% for the lateral incisor/central incisor and 84% for the canine/lateral incisor. Forster and colleagues[9] reported that the average tooth to tooth width proportion of patients evaluated at a

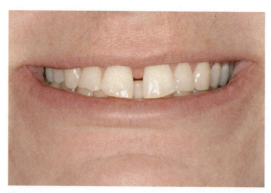

Fig. 2. Smile with diastema.

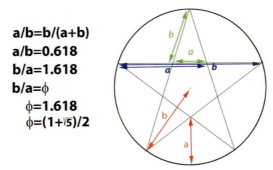

$a/b = b/(a+b)$
$a/b = 0.618$
$b/a = 1.618$
$b/a = \phi$
$\phi = 1.618$
$\phi = (1+\sqrt{5})/2$

Fig. 3. The golden proportion.

faculty of dentistry in Hungary was 62% for the lateral incisor/central incisor and 85% for the canine/lateral incisor. Asians often report lateral incisors that are smaller than their North American and European counterparts. When reviewing articles to understand the natural proportions that exist, it is important to consider the ethnicity and region in which the study was performed to determine their applicability when designing smiles in other areas of the world.

The average width/length (w/l) ratio of the maxillary central incisor has been reported in one well-known study to be 85% to 86%.[10] Another study reports the mean w/l ratio of the central incisor to be 90%.[11] The w/l ratio can be influenced by several factors. Most studies evaluate the visible display of the length of the central incisor, not the distance from the incisal edge to the cementoenamel junction. Altered passive eruption in young patients who are often evaluated in studies would result in a higher reported observed w/l ratio than if the entire clinical crown were exposed.[12] As a patient ages, there can be incisal wear that also increases the w/l ratio.[13] Age variations can be a significant factor affecting the w/l ratio values reported. **Fig. 4** is an imaged photograph of a natural proportion smile with the Preston width proportion (66%, 84%) and the 86% w/l ratio of the central incisor.

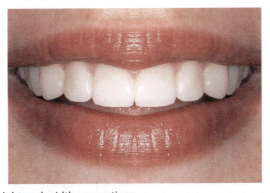

Fig. 4. Natural height and width proportions.

RECURRING ESTHETIC DENTAL PROPORTION

The recurring esthetic dental (RED) proportion has been proposed as a model in designing smiles.[14] The RED proportion states that the proportion of the successive widths of the teeth as viewed from the front should remain constant as one moves distally (**Fig. 5**). The frontal view width of every maxillary tooth becomes smaller by a certain percentage as one moves posteriorly. This is a two-dimensional evaluation of a three-dimensional smile, so the buccal/palatal placement of the teeth affects their apparent widths. The range of suggested RED proportions is between 62% and 80%. The golden proportion (62% RED proportion) is applicable as one of many proportions that fit within the definition of the RED proportion. Different RED proportions can be proposed for use with the same individual according to the desired length of the teeth, the scope of treatment possible, and the desire to have the size of the teeth match the size of the face and body (**Fig. 6**). The expanded definition of the RED proportion includes using the relative tooth height and body height to determine the appropriate RED proportion.

PREFERRED PROPORTIONS VERSUS NATURAL PROPORTIONS

A study comparing different RED proportions with different heights of teeth found dentists surveyed preferred a resulting smile that kept the w/l ratio of the resulting central incisor in the 75% to 78% range.[15] Dentists surveyed preferred people with tall teeth to have a wider central incisor to maintain the preferred 75% to 78% w/l ratio. This is different than the 85% to 86% w/l ratio, which has been reported as what is observed in natural teeth (**Fig. 7**). Another study comparing different proposed and natural tooth to tooth width proportions found that a slight majority of dentists surveyed preferred the 70% RED proportion to the Preston proportion with normal-length teeth.[16] Most dentists surveyed preferred proportions that are not coincident with natural proportions. This asks the question whether naturally occurring proportions should always be used when patient elective treatment is sought. **Fig. 8** is an imaged photograph of a smile with the 70% RED proportion and the 78% w/l ratio of the central incisor.

AFFECT OF CENTRAL INCISOR HEIGHT ON CENTRAL INCISOR WIDTH AND APPROPRIATE RECURRING ESTHETIC DENTAL PROPORTION

Because the preferred maxillary central incisors of tall teeth are also wider they occupy a greater percentage of the smile leaving less space for the remaining anterior teeth (**Fig. 9**). The width of the lateral incisors and canines must be a smaller percentage of the central incisor resulting in a smaller RED proportion being preferred. The smaller the RED proportion, the more dominant is the central incisor. Smiles designed using

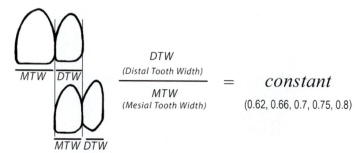

Fig. 5. RED proportion formula. (*Adapted from* Ward DH. Proportional smile design using the recurring esthetic dental proportion. Dent Clin North Am 2001;45:146; with permission.)

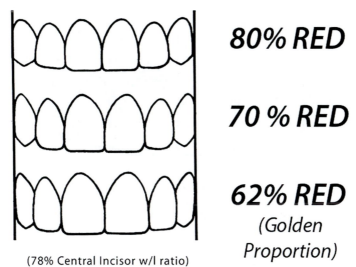

80% RED

70 % RED

62% RED
(Golden Proportion)

(78% Central Incisor w/l ratio)

Fig. 6. RED proportions.

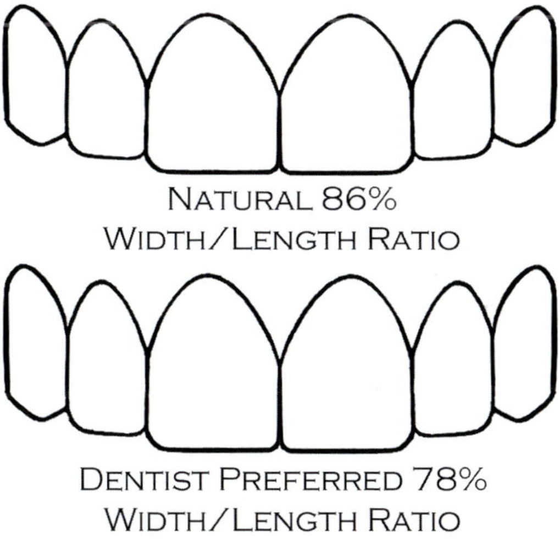

NATURAL 86%
WIDTH/LENGTH RATIO

DENTIST PREFERRED 78%
WIDTH/LENGTH RATIO

Fig. 7. Natural versus preferred width/length ratio.

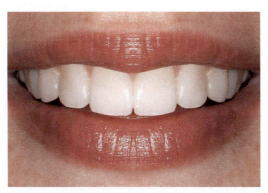

Fig. 8. 70% RED proportion, 78% width/length ratio.

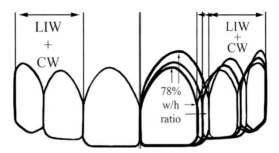

Less Remaining Width for Lateral and Canine

Fig. 9. Taller tooth yields more dominant central incisor. CW, canine width; LIW, lateral incisor width. (*Adapted from* Ward DH. Using the RED proportion to engineer the perfect smile. Dent Today 2008;27(5):112; with permission.)

the golden proportion (62% RED) exhibit prominent central incisors, which together occupy 50% of the intercanine width (ICW). This seems logical when one considers that tall models tend to look more attractive with smiles designed with the 62% RED (golden) proportion. Conversely, dentists preferred people with short teeth to have more narrow central incisors to maintain the preferred 75% to 78% w/l ratio. Because the central incisors do not occupy as much space there is more room for the remaining anterior teeth and the lateral incisors and canines are more similar in width resulting in a larger RED proportion (**Fig. 10**). The percentage difference is not as great as one moves distally, resulting in a RED proportion closer to 80%.

CORRELATING THE TOOTH AND BODY HEIGHT WITH THE RECURRING ESTHETIC DENTAL PROPORTION

It is recommended that the taller the individual and taller the teeth, the smaller the RED proportion. Extra tall individuals should have a 62% RED proportion, normal height persons a 70% RED proportion, and a very short person an 80% RED proportion. Interpolations should be used within these parameters for medium tall and medium short individuals (**Fig. 11**). These are guidelines that should take into account the preoperative conditions of the teeth.

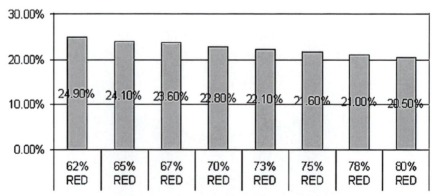

Fig. 10. Central incisor width percentage of intercanine width for different RED proportions.

Different RED Proportions
(Central Incisor 78% w/l ratio)   Tooth Length

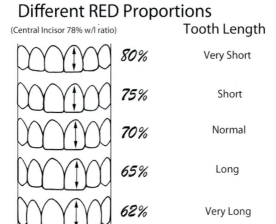

80%	Very Short
75%	Short
70%	Normal
65%	Long
62%	Very Long

Fig. 11. RED proportions correlating to tooth length. (*Adapted from* Ward DH. Using the RED proportion template to create a beautiful smile. Oral Health 2014;104(4):103; with permission.)

COMPARING NORMAL HEIGHT 70% RECURRING ESTHETIC DENTAL PROPORTION SMILES WITH PRESTON NATURAL PROPORTIONS

When comparing norms as determined by Preston, the resulting width of the central incisor was nearly identical to the width as determined using the 70% RED proportion. The lateral incisor, however, was wider (70% the central incisor width [CIW]) when using the RED proportion compared with what was found in the population (66% the CIW). The canine was narrower (70% the lateral incisor width [LIW]) when using the RED proportion than when compared with the general population (84% the LIW) (**Fig. 12**).

USING THE RECURRING ESTHETIC DENTAL PROPORTION

When using the RED proportion, the ICW is used to determine the ideal width of the central incisor. The formula for determining the ideal width of the central incisor is $CIW = ICW/2 (1+RED+RED^2)$. Substituting 0.7 for the RED value into the equation one finds that with normal-length teeth you divide the ICW by 4.38 to calculate the width of the central incisor (**Fig. 13**). The LIW is determined by multiplying the CIW times the RED proportion. The canine width is determined by multiplying the resulting

Preston Proportion

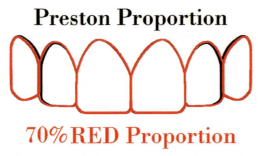

70% RED Proportion

Fig. 12. Comparing Preston with RED proportion (normal length teeth). (*Adapted from* Ward DH. A study of dentists' preferred maxillary anterior tooth width proportions: comparing the recurring esthetic dental proportion to other mathematical and naturally occurring proportions. J Esthet Restor Dent 2007;19:330; with permission.)

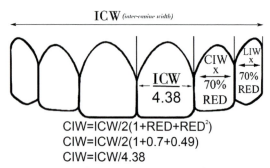

$$CIW=ICW/2(1+RED+RED^2)$$
$$CIW=ICW/2(1+0.7+0.49)$$
$$CIW=ICW/4.38$$

Fig. 13. Using RED proportion to determine tooth widths for normal length teeth CIW to ICW. (*Adapted from* Ward DH. Using the RED proportion to engineer the perfect smile. Dent Today 2008;27(5):114; with permission.)

LIW times the RED proportion. **Table 1** calculates tooth widths from relative tooth heights using the RED proportion and ICW.

For any given ICW there are several RED proportions that can be used. Body type, facial/skeletal form, lip form, gingival display, and tooth display should all be considered. Creating a smile that is coincident with the proportions of the body type dictates that a very tall person would have a smile with a 62% RED proportion, an average height person a 70% RED proportion, and a very short person an 80% RED proportion. The smile created using these proportions is quite different and yet all can be pleasing especially if they match the body type of the patient (**Fig. 14**).

SIMPLIFIED METHOD OF CALCULATING THE TOOTH DIMENSIONS USING THE RECURRING ESTHETIC DENTAL PROPORTION

A simplified method has been developed for determining the size of the maxillary anterior teeth using the RED proportion. If one substitutes the 78% w/l ratio into the formula and solves the equations for different height teeth one can use a chart to look up the appropriate widths of the anterior teeth. The first step is to measure the facial view intercommissural width of the anterior six teeth and divide it by the length of the central incisor. The resulting product is looked up in the chart and the intercommissural width is divided by the appropriate numbers in the chart to determine the widths of the central incisor, lateral incisor, and canine (**Table 2**).

Table 1
Calculating the RED proportion and anterior total widths from ICW with different tooth heights

Desired RED Proportion		Intercanine Divisors (Rounded): ICW/(N) = Tooth Width		
Tooth Height	RED Proportion	Central Incisor Width	Lateral Incisor Width	Canine Width
Very tall	62% RED	ICW/4.0	CIW *0.62	LIW ×0.62
Tall	66% RED	ICW/4.2	CIW *0.66	LIW ×0.66
Normal	70% RED	ICW/4.4	CIW *0.7	LIW ×0.7
Short	75% RED	ICW/4.6	CIW *0.75	LIW ×0.75
Very short	80% RED	ICW/4.8	CIW *0.8	LIW ×0.8

Adapted from Ward DH. Using the RED proportion to engineer the perfect smile. Dent Today 2008;27(5):116; with permission.

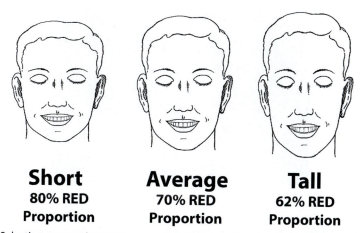

Fig. 14. Selecting appropriate RED proportion that coordinates with the body/tooth height.

The length of the central incisor is determined by dividing the width of the central incisor by 0.78. If a change in the length of the central incisor is desired, the Inter-canine Width (ICW) can be divided by the desired Central Incisor Length (CIL). This quotient should be between 3.1 and 3.8. and looked up in the left column of **Table 2** to determine the appropriate RED Proportion. The row with the RED Proportion is used to determine how to calculate the corresponding central incisor width, lateral incisor width and canine width.

USE OF DIGITAL IMAGING

Digital imaging is an invaluable tool in demonstrating to the patient the possible outcomes using different RED proportions and width/length ratios and can help them make informed decisions regarding additional procedures and the extensiveness of the prosthetic restoration. Patients are often reluctant to undergo additional surgical procedures but may be more willing to proceed if they can see the potential outcomes of their treatment decisions. A patient with short clinical crowns was interested in improving her smile. Photographs were taken (**Fig. 15**). A template with outlines of the anterior teeth with different RED proportions was moved over the smile

Table 2
Simplified method of determining anterior tooth widths from ICW and CIH

ICW/CIH	RED Proportion	Central Incisor Width (ICW/N)	Lateral Incisor Width (ICW/N)	Canine Width (ICW/N)
3.1	62% RED	4.00	6.47	10.43
3.2	65% RED	4.15	6.38	9.81
3.3	67% RED	4.24	6.33	9.44
3.4	70% RED	4.38	6.26	8.94
3.5	73% RED	4.53	6.20	8.49
3.6	75% RED	4.63	6.17	8.22
3.7	78% RED	4.78	6.12	7.85
3.8	80% RED	4.88	6.10	7.63

Abbreviation: CIH, central incisor height.
Adapted from Ward DH. Using the RED proportion to engineer the perfect smile. Dent Today 2008;27(5):116; with permission.

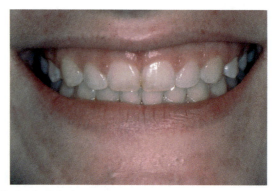

Fig. 15. Smile with short clinical crowns.

photograph to help evaluate the proportions and to select an appropriate RED proportion (**Fig. 16**). The 80% RED proportion was selected and the 80% template superimposed over the photograph (**Fig. 17**). An imaged photograph was produced to show the potential affect of crown lengthening and laminates (**Fig. 18**). Imaging is a powerful and effective way to communicate with patients, specialists, and the dental laboratory.

DETERMINING THE IDEAL WIDTH AND LENGTH OF THE CENTRAL INCISOR USING THE RECURRING ESTHETIC DENTAL PROPORTION

The RED proportion mathematical formulas can be useful to determine the width and length of the ideal central incisor. Using the 70% RED proportion calculations also results in a reliable way to determine the widths of the central incisors observed in nature as reported by Preston. Whether the RED proportion is used or not for the

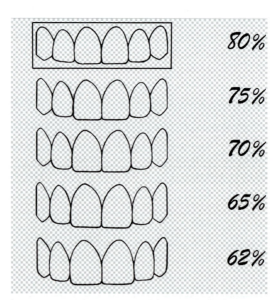

Fig. 16. Template chosen to superimpose over photograph. (*Adapted from* Ward DH. Using the RED proportion template to create a beautiful smile. Oral Health 2014;104(4):103; with permission.)

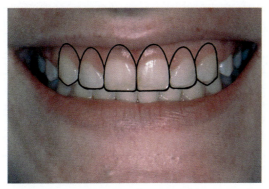

Fig. 17. Smile with 80% RED proportion template overlaid.

determination of the width of the lateral incisors is up to the dentist and the patient. It has been advocated with denture making, that variations of the lateral incisor in position and alignment help to give individuality to a smile. Some believe that a narrow lateral incisor is considered to be a more feminine trait, although this fact cannot be proved in studies of natural teeth.[17,18] If a narrower lateral incisor is used, then a wider canine is necessary. This seems to be the case in nature. **Table 3** is a simplified method to determine the ideal width and length of the central incisor using the principles of the RED proportion.

PREFERRED SMILE PROPORTIONS

Studies have been performed to determine the proportions most pleasing to dentists and patients. Generally patient preferences vary widely and are not as selective as those of dentists.[19,20] If dentists who are more particular about esthetic smiles are pleased, then it is hoped that in most instances the patient will also be satisfied. However, smile preferences can also be subjective. Patients should be shown the potential look of the smile before active treatment is commenced. Once approved this photograph should be conveyed to the specialists and the dental laboratory.

CASE STUDY

A 58-year-old man presented to the office unhappy with his smile. He had not been in a dental office for several years. A complete examination was performed, radiographs

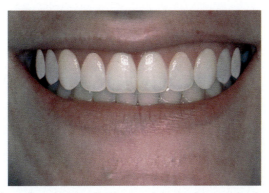

Fig. 18. Imaged view of potential smile if crown lengthening and laminates are placed.

Table 3
Calculating CIL and CIW from ICW with different tooth heights

| Tooth Height | Desired RED Proportion | | |
	RED Proportion	CIW	CIL
Very tall	62% RED	ICW/4	ICW/3.1
Tall	66% RED	ICW/4.2	ICW/3.25
Normal	70% RED	ICW/4.4	ICW/3.4
Short	75% RED	ICW/4.6	ICW/3.6
Very short	80% RED	ICW/4.8	ICW/3.8

Abbreviation: CIL, central incisor length.

exposed, and photographs taken (**Fig. 19**). There was a lack of posterior occlusion and the bite had collapsed. The patient was a musician who played a brass instrument. He wanted to keep his anterior teeth so his embouchure would remain intact.

The sizes of the teeth were evaluated. The intercommisural width measured 39.2 mm as viewed from the front (**Fig. 20**). It was determined that normal-length teeth were desired to match his dentition and his body type. Looking in **Table 3** for normal-length teeth the central incisor length is determined by dividing the ICW by 3.4, which was 11.5 mm (**Fig. 21**). The 70% RED proportion template was superimposed over the preoperative photograph to give an idea of the relative size of the desired anterior teeth (**Fig. 22**).

Unrestorable posterior teeth were extracted. The maxillary anterior teeth were restored with composite to give an idea of how the final restorations would look. This allowed us to see if the patient could accommodate the position of the incisal edges and if he could perform properly on his brass instrument (**Fig. 23**). Interim partial prostheses were fabricated to determine the proper vertical dimension of occlusion. The patient was allowed 6 months to adjust to the occlusion.

The maxillary anterior teeth were prepared for crowns and provisional restorations fabricated (**Fig. 24**). The laboratory was sent models and photographs of the provisional restorations. The crowns were fabricated by the laboratory, tried in, and seated (**Fig. 25**). The patient was thrilled with his new smile and his ability to play his instrument.

Treatment for this patient is not complete. He had three maxillary and three mandibular implants placed on his right side. Custom abutments were fabricated and crowns were seated (**Fig. 26**). Future plans include restoring his left side.

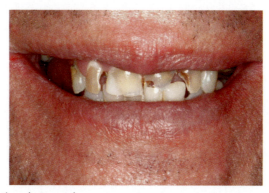

Fig. 19. Preoperative photograph.

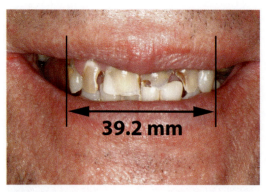

Fig. 20. Measuring ICW.

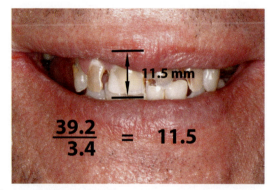

Fig. 21. Calculating central incisor length.

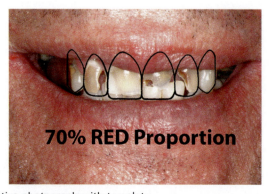

Fig. 22. Preoperative photograph with template.

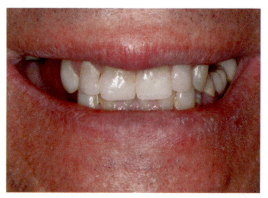

Fig. 23. Anterior teeth built to desired size in composite.

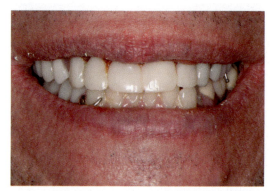

Fig. 24. Anterior teeth prepared and provisionalized. Posterior teeth replaced with interim removable prostheses.

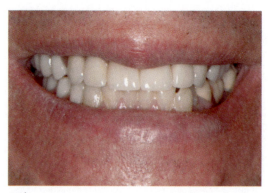

Fig. 25. Crowns seated.

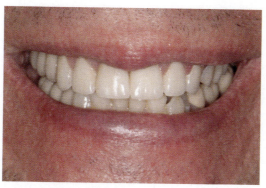

Fig. 26. Anterior teeth and right side restored.

SUMMARY

Smile design should include evaluation of the body, face, and existing dentition of the patient. The RED proportion is a useful tool in designing a smile that is in sync with the size of the individual. Although not readily observed in nature, these methods can be useful when designing smiles.

REFERENCES

1. Chu SJ. Range and mean distribution frequency of individual tooth widths of the maxillary anterior dentition. Pract Proced Aesthet Dent 2007;19(4):209–15.
2. Fayyad MA, Jamani KD, Aqrabawi J. Geometric and mathematical proportions and their relations to maxillary anterior teeth. J Contemp Dent Pract 2006;7(5): 62–70.
3. Levin EI. Dental esthetics and the golden proportion. J Prosthet Dent 1978;40: 244–52.
4. Rufenacht CR. Fundamentals of esthetics. Chicago: Quintessence; 1990. p. 67–134.
5. Huntley HE. The divine proportion: a study in mathematical beauty. New York: Dover Publications Inc; 1970.
6. Hasanreisoglu U, Berksun S, Aras K, et al. An Analysis of maxillary anterior teeth: facial and dental proportions. J Prosthet Dent 2005;94:530–8.
7. Mahsid M, Khoshvaghti A, Varshosaz M, et al. Evaluation of "golden proportion" in individuals with an esthetic smile. J Esthet Restor Dent 2004;16:185–92.
8. Preston JD. The golden proportion revisited. J Esthet Dent 1993;5:247–51.
9. Forster A, Velez R, Antal M, et al. Width ratios in the anterior maxillary region in a Hungarian population: addition to the golden proportion debate. J Prosthet Dent 2013;110:211–5.
10. Sterrett JD, Oliver T, Robinson F, et al. Width/length ratios of normal clinical crowns of the maxillary anterior dentition in man. J Clin Periodontol 1999;26: 153–7.
11. Gillen RJ, Schwartz RS, Hilton TJ, et al. An analysis of selected normative tooth proportions. Int J Prosthodont 1994;7:410–7.
12. Rossi R, Benedetti R, Santos-Morales RI. Treatment of altered passive eruption: periodontal plastic surgery of the dentogingival junction. Eur J Esthet Dent 2008;3:212–23.

13. Magne P, Gallucci GO, Belser UC. Anatomical crown width/length ratios of un-worn and worn maxillary teeth in white subjects. J Prosthet Dent 2003;89:453–61.
14. Ward DH. Proportional smile design using the RED proportion. Dent Clin North Am 2001;45:143–54.
15. Rosenstiel SF, Ward DH, Rashid RG. Dentists' preferences of anterior tooth pro-portion: a web-based study. J Prosthodont 2000;9:123–36.
16. Ward DH. A study of dentists' preferred maxillary anterior tooth width proportions: comparing the recurring esthetic dental proportion to other mathematical and naturally occurring proportions. J Esthet Restor Dent 2007;19:323–36.
17. Lombardi RE. A method for the classification of errors in dental esthetics. J Prosthet Dent 1974;32:501–13.
18. Basting RT, Trindale RS, Flório FM. Comparative study of smile analysis by sub-jective and computerized methods. Oper Dent 2006;31:652–9.
19. Ker AJ, Chan R, Fields HW, et al. Esthetics and smile characteristics from the lay-person's perspective: a computer-based survey study. J Am Dent Assoc 2008; 139(10):1318–27.
20. Rosenstiel SF, Rashid RG. Public preferences for anterior tooth variations. J Esthet Restor Dent 2002;14:97–106.

Cosmetic Makeover
Ensuring Patient Input in a
Multidisciplinary Treatment

Sabrina Magid-Katz, DMD[a],*, Kenneth S. Magid, DDS, FICD[a],
Theo Mantzikos, DDS[b]

KEYWORDS

- Cosmetic makeover • Multidisciplinary • Patient input • Predicable results

KEY POINTS

- A cosmetic smile makeover is a sought after procedure in our esthetically driven society, requiring participation of dental specialists, restorative dentists, and laboratory technicians.
- To promote patient satisfaction, all involved parties, including the patient, must be aware of the results that can be achieved and what it will require to achieve them.
- Although treatment can be redone, it cannot be undone; therefore, it is wise to solicit and consider patient input before treatment and before the final restorations are cemented.

INTRODUCTION

In practicing "cosmetic dentistry," the dentist is often presented with a patient whose desire for esthetic improvement of their smile is mitigated by the fear of loss of control, and the unknown happiness with the final outcome. These concerns are beyond the simple reassurance by the dentist that "everything will turn out beautiful in the end." During the consultation and before case acceptance, the dentist often shows the patient photographs of other cosmetic cases in an effort to convince the patient of their skill and talent. This, however, does not alter the patient's concerns about whether they will be happy with their result. In addition, the dentist is faced with the possibility that the patient's preconceived vision of a desirable outcome will not coincide with the dentist's case-based restorative design. The dentist's greatest fear should be that in the end and after measurably successful treatment, the patient may not be satisfied. This unfortunate result is a distinct possibility when the sequence of treatment is tooth preparation followed by temporary restorations that either conform to the original teeth, are generic in size and shape, or are nonpredictive of

The authors have nothing to disclose.
[a] Department of Cariology and Comprehensive Care, NYU College of Dentistry, New York, NY 10010, USA; [b] Private Practice, White Plains, NY, USA
* Corresponding author.
E-mail address: sbm236@nyu.edu

Dent Clin N Am 59 (2015) 639–645
http://dx.doi.org/10.1016/j.cden.2015.03.009
dental.theclinics.com

the final restorations. This treatment leaves the design of the final restorations completely in the hands of the ceramist, without input from the dentist or patient. With this treatment scenario the first time the patient sees their final smile they are bonded into place and they are handed a mirror. Fait accompli.

These difficulties are further exacerbated in a clinical presentation with desires for change that are not possible through restorative treatment alone. In these cases, consultation with other specialists must be a part of the initial workup to determine in advance the restorative plan and what the final outcome will be.

This case report takes a different approach to cosmetic treatment that ensures full communication between restorative dentist, dental specialists, laboratory ceramist, and, most important, the patient. Because the final result is never in doubt, both a happy patient and a happy dentist can be assured. As Steven Covey says in 7 Habits of Highly Successful People, "Begin with the end in mind."[1]

Case Presentation

The patient, a 42-year-old Caucasian female, presented with a chief complaint of unhappiness with her smile (**Fig. 1**). Consultation with the patient revealed apprehension about the result being natural in appearance and beautiful. The patient was assured that there would be no unhappy surprises as, using the method described herein, she would have input into every step of the process.

The cosmetic process began with a series of photographs, study models, digital radiographs, and completion of the NYU College of Dentistry Smile Evaluation Form. Evaluation of these records revealed no active caries and the presence of class III and class V restorations that would not interfere with treatment. The maxillary

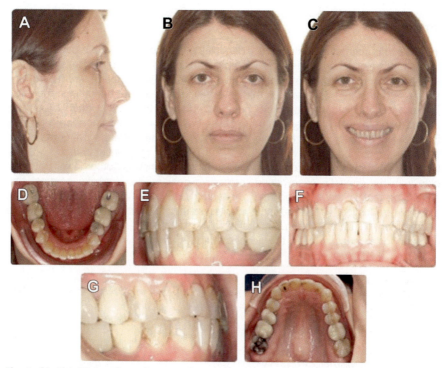

Fig. 1. (A–H) Initial patient photographs.

incisors were considerably worn and the lower incisors supererupted and in an edge-to-edge relationship with the maxillary teeth. The complete analysis indicated that orthodontic intervention would be necessary, followed by modification of the soft tissue surrounding the teeth to provide proper gingival heights and zenith points.

The initial photographs and models were shared with the orthodontist to determine the amount of movement that could be expected and the amount of clearance for the final restorations. This team approach is essential before developing any cosmetic plan to avoid an unrealistic and unachievable preview. A potential cosmetic design was determined using the orthodontist's input, and guidelines developed for the optimal design of the dental smile. The "golden percentage"[2] was used to determine the desired width of each of the teeth in the esthetic zone based on the full cuspid-to-cuspid distance when viewed from the facial aspect. Once the width was determined the position of the central incisors was established based on the reveal of the incisal edge at rest and its anterior–posterior location at the wet–dry line of the lip. It was necessary to ensure that this position fall within the interarch clearance that could be provided by the orthodontic movement. Using the width of the central incisor the length was determined using the ratio of 0.8/1 and the smile line established based on the central incisor position and the curvature of the lower lip during smiling. All of this information was put together as a proposed cosmetic design and sent for a computerized cosmetic preview (DaVinci Dental Laboratories; **Fig. 2**).

The computerized preview offers the advantage of allowing the patient to view the cosmetic changes that can be effected. At this point in the process, it would be impossible for the patient to preview the potential alterations by any other means. The

A   **B**

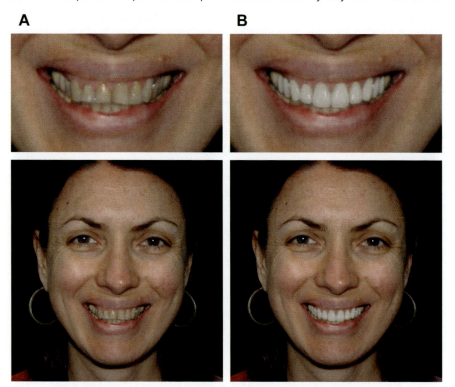

Fig. 2. (*A–B*) Computerized cosmetic preview based on an analysis of the dentition and proposed treatment.

potential hazard of this technique is to show changes that are, in fact, not possible clinically. Although a disclaimer is often shown on the bottom of these photographs, showing a patient changes that cannot be accomplished defeats the purpose of this communication and can lead to a very dissatisfied patient. The dentist using this technology must always do so with a firm clinical grasp of what can be accomplished and remain within those constraints.

The preview image was shown to the patient during a second consultation. This viewing affords the patient their first opportunity to see the proposed treatment result and opens a full discussion of their likes and dislikes. The size and shape of the teeth, the tooth color, tooth display while smiling, and incisal edge position are reviewed. It is a great advantage to have a computer program in the office that allows slight modification of the preview during this phase of consultation. For comparison, changes can be made, at the patient's request, to 1 side of the smile. As the patient watches, they are drawn into the process. Once the patient is happy with the previewed result, the actual clinical phase of treatment was begun. It is important to realize that at this point the dentist and the patient both know where the final treatment will be taking them, while at the same time nothing irreversible had been done.

TREATMENT SEQUENCE
Orthodontic Considerations

The interdisiciplinary orthodontic treatment plan required the establishment of a favorable alignment of the bimaxillary anterior dentition with improvement in the overbite/overjet relationship. Consultation with the restorative dentist provided information about the desired incisal edge position of the final restorations and the amount of clearance needed from the lower incisors. In this particular case, it was felt particular attention should be paid that the final outcome provided cuspid guidance so as to protect the anterior and posterior dentition (**Fig. 3**).

Orthodontic treatment was initiated utilizing clear, active removable appliances (Invisalign) for the primary level and alignment of the anterior dentition and establishing the most favorable anterior dental position. Favorable alignment of the bimaxillary anterior dentition was achieved with Invisalign, but limitations in the ability to control intrusive/extrusive movements of the anterior dentition were recognized. Consequently, conversion to esthetic fixed orthodontic appliances (ceramic braces) was pursued.

Fixed ceramic orthodontic brackets were placed on the maxillary and mandibular dentition (first premolar to first premolar) in coordination with an 0.016 nickel titanium archwire for further ideal level and alignment of the dentition. In subsequent appointments intervals, the archwire was upgraded to a .017 × .025 stainless steel allowing for individual torque/vertical bends, along with bracket repositioning, to accommodate the axial inclinations that would be required for restorative preparation of the underlying dentition.

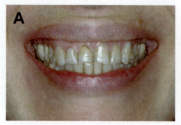 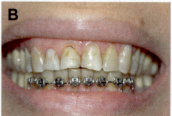

Fig. 3. Evaluation showing (A) before and after (B) initial orthodontic phase.

Once the dental position was confirmed as consistent with the esthetic dental treatment to be performed, the ceramic brackets were removed and immediate insertion of clear, removable retaining appliances were provided to maintain the dentition.

The final orthodontic result allowed for favorable alignment of the dentition, orthodontic stability, and a favorable anterior dental relationship in anticipation of the perioprosthetic esthetic enhancement.

Restorative Design

A new series of photographs and study models was taken and a Kois dentofacial analyzer was used to mount the case on a Panadent articulator. The initial cosmetic design, which was established before treatment, was evaluated based on the realities of the orthodontic result. This design and the initial pretreatment computer preview were sent to the ceramists's laboratory for a final cosmetic wax up (**Fig. 4**). A consultation with the patient using the initial computerized cosmetic preview, which she had approved, and the proposed final wax up, put the patient's mind at ease that; as we had promised, we were indeed using her input and giving her some control of the final outcome. Although not necessary in this case, we will often use the wax up to create a putty stent, which is filled with a flowable composite (Luxatemp DMG) and placed over the patient's teeth. This technique does not show tooth structure or soft tissue that must be removed for the final result, but it does give the patient an idea of the result in their mouth. Once the patient approves the "mock up," the composite is easily removed.

Periodontal Considerations

Once orthodontic movement of the teeth was completed providing sufficient horizontal overjet and vertical clearance for correct incisal edge positioning, the soft tissue contours were evaluated. A clear stent fabricated on a duplicate of the wax up was used to determine the final gingival positions. Evaluating the changes necessary and periodontal probing ensured that we would only be affecting soft tissue and that the biologic width would not be invaded.

Restorative Sequence

The patient was anesthetized and minor correction of the gingival zenith height and shape was accomplished using a diode laser at 550°C with thermal feedback (Dental Photonics). Teeth #4 through #13 were prepared for feldspathic porcelain veneers. Because there is minimal collateral thermal damage and no visible recession using a temperature-controlled diode laser,[3,4] the procedure was performed at the same visit as veneer preparation and impression. An incisal guide created on the wax up

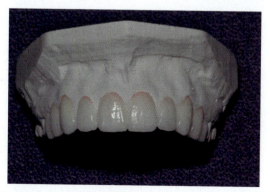

Fig. 4. Esthetic wax up on a prepared model.

was used to ensure sufficient reduction of the tooth structure and position of the incisal edges. This step is critical to avoid the common problem of pronation of the final restorations due to insufficient clearance.

After impressions the teeth were temporized using Luxatemp (DMG) in a putty matrix of the wax up (**Fig. 5**). This step transfers the photographic alteration and the patient approved wax up to the patient's mouth. The patient and dentist can now preview the final result as it will actually appear and make any changes necessary to the easily modified composite material.

The patient returned 2 days later after living with the cosmetic changes and having gotten the opinion of those important to her. Had the patient wanted modification of the temporary restorations, those changes would have been easily made using fine diamonds and flowable composite. Changes can be made to 1 side of the smile and the patient can observe the alterations by looking left and right to determine which side they prefer. The patient would then be sent home to live with the modified temporary restorations and brought back for approval. This can be done as many times as is necessary until the desired result is achieved. Although sometimes frustrating, this technique is a far better method of dealing with changes than once the final porcelain has been inserted.

In the case presented here, the patient was extremely happy with the resulting appearance and form of the temporaries and no changes were required. Using the color of the temporaries as a baseline, she participated in the shade selection of the final restorations. Additional photographs and models were taken and provided to the ceramist (Jason Kim, Oral Design New York) to guide the production of the final veneers. When the veneers were returned to the office, they were placed on the model and measurement comparisons were taken to ensure that they corresponded with the model of the temporary restorations that the patient had approved. Although slight differences and improvements of the contours and surface are normally found, this check avoids the ceramist making changes in tooth position or shape that may not be approved by the patient.

Insertion Visit

After removing the temporaries the final feldspathic veneers were tried in with water for the patient's approval. This very last step in the process gives the patient the final control over whether the veneers are irreversibly bonded into place. Additionally, this is an important psychological step in having the patient be comfortable with the process. Using a standard isolation protocol, the veneers were then bonded into place (**Fig. 6**).

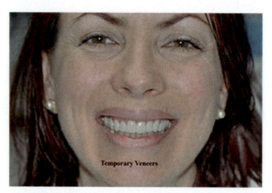

Fig. 5. Temporary veneers in place for patient evaluation.

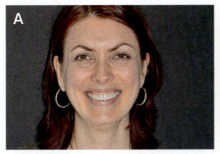 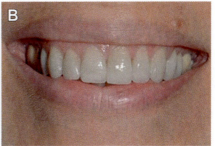

Fig. 6. (*A*) Final patient smile. (*B*) Close up of final smile.

The patient returned to the office 2 days after insertion to make any final adjustments. At this time, the anesthetic had worn off and she had had the opportunity to "live with" the restorations. The final result was just as she had expected based on the initial cosmetic preview, the wax up, and the temporary restorations. We, as well as the patient were extremely pleased with management and outcome of this case.

SUMMARY

Ensuring that there are no "unhappy surprises" is of prime importance to patients and dentists. This procedure outlines the steps necessary to provide both the dentist and the patient complete control of a smile makeover even in a difficult multidisciplinary case.

REFERENCES

1. Covey S. 7 habits of highly successful people. Free Press; 1989.
2. Snow S. Esthetic smile analysis of maxillary anterior tooth width: the golden percentage. J Esthet Dent 1999;11:177–84.
3. Magid K. Presentation to Academy of Laser Dentistry based upon research done by dental photonics. 2011.
4. Magid K, Strauss R. Laser use for esthetic soft tissue modification. Dent Clin North Am 2007;51:525–45.

Esthetic Correction of Orthodontically Transposed Teeth with Veneers and Laser Periodontal Modification

Kenneth S. Magid, DDS, FICD[a],*, Zahid Juma, DDS[b]

KEYWORDS

• Orthodontically transposed teeth • Veneers • Laser crown lengthening

KEY POINTS

- Missing teeth in the esthetic zone, whether congenital or as a result of other factors, present difficult choices in clinical management.
- The missing teeth can be replaced by surgical or restorative intervention but are often treated orthodontically.
- These repositioned teeth often lead to an unaesthetic result because of differences in morphology, color, and particularly in gingival architecture.
- The use of multiple lasers for periodontal modification and feldspathic porcelain veneers can help achieve a highly esthetic result.

INTRODUCTION

Dentists are frequently presented with the problem of missing teeth in the esthetic zone, whether caused by disease or trauma or they are congenitally missing. Most frequently this occurs with one or more lateral incisors but any of the anterior teeth can be affected. In adult patients, this is most often treated by placing an implant-supported restoration. Alternatively, a prosthetic replacement is chosen, such as a full-coverage supported fixed bridge or a pontic supported by one or more bonded retainers.

For adolescent patients, the decision may be made to move the teeth orthodontically to close the space. Although orthodontic treatment will be successful in closing

---

The authors have nothing to disclose.
[a] Department of Cariology and Comprehensive Care, NYU College of Dentistry, New York, New York 10010, USA; [b] Coast Dental in Deland, 237 E international Speedway Blvd, Suite 1B, DeLand, FL 32720, USA
* Corresponding author.
E-mail address: ken.magid@gmail.com

Dent Clin N Am 59 (2015) 647–654
http://dx.doi.org/10.1016/j.cden.2015.03.005
0011-8532/15/$ – see front matter © 2015 Elsevier Inc. All rights reserved.

the space left by the missing teeth, it is less successful in providing a truly esthetic result. Each tooth in the esthetic zone has a specific morphology and is very different in size and shape from its neighbors. This unique morphology is obvious in appearance and also has a different emergence profile from the tooth normally in that position, which results in gingival heights and contours that are unharmonious and unaesthetic.

When the restorative dentist is presented with the challenge of providing an esthetic makeover under these circumstances, it is important to deal not only with the teeth but also with the periodontal tissues. A complete periodontal evaluation is necessary to determine if the correction needed involves only the soft tissue or if osseous recontouring is necessary to achieve the desired result. Although osseous surgery can be affected by traditional means, such as scalpel and open flap surgery, advances in dental lasers have provided an alternative that has many advantages. The laser procedures are done without the problem of bleeding that hides the operative field and without the necessity for sutures. The use of lasers for periodontal modification also provides a predictable result that is essential in creating optimal esthetics.

CASE PRESENTATION

The patient is a man in his early 20s endeavoring to be an actor. He presented to the honors esthetics clinic at the New York University (NYU) College of Dentistry complaining that he did not like the shape and color of his teeth. The examination revealed that a congenitally missing tooth No. 8 had been previously treated by orthodontically moving No. 7 to the No. 8 position, No. 6 to the No. 7 position, and No. 5 to the No. 6 position and the remaining teeth on the right side moved anteriorly to eliminate the resulting space. Although this treatment provided a fully dentate arch, it did not compensate for the discrepancy in shape, color, or gingival architecture between the newly positioned teeth and the contralateral arch (**Figs. 1** and **2**). To evaluate the patient and determine the treatment necessary, an American Academy of Cosmetic Dentistry series of photographs, full series of radiographs, periodontal probing, and study models were taken; and an NYU College of Dentistry Esthetic Evaluation Form was completed.

PERIODONTAL CONSIDERATIONS

Evaluation of the tissues surrounding the teeth revealed a significant discrepancy in the gingival height and shape (**Fig. 3**A). Full periodontal charting was within normal limits and indicated that the desired changes to the periodontal tissue of teeth No.

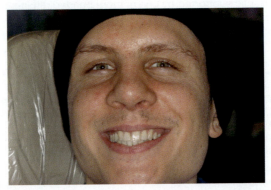

Fig. 1. Full-face photograph showing unaesthetic appearance of the smile.

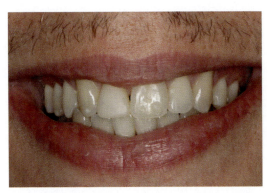

Fig. 2. Close-up view making apparent the discrepancy between right and left sides as a result of different color and morphology of the teeth and unbalanced arch form.

5 and No. 7 would invade the biological width (see **Fig. 3**B, perio chart). If this was not dealt with by osseous surgery to restore appropriate architecture, the result could be chronic inflammatory disease in the area or uncontrolled recession depending on the tissue type. Measurement of the attached gingiva indicated sufficient tissue for periodontal alteration and the necessity to move the maxillary frenum attachment by frenectomy. This correction could be accomplished using scalpel reshaping and full-flap osseous contouring; but it was decided instead to use multiple laser wavelengths in a flapless technique, which would require no suturing and a shorter overall healing interval. The erbium laser has been shown to be effective in osseous recontouring with no collateral tissue damage and comparable healing with other methods.[1]

RESTORATIVE CONSIDERATIONS

Because the teeth that were moved into positions 6, 7, and 8 had very different morphology from those on the contralateral side, preparation for the proposed feldspathic veneers would necessitate a more difficult process than the standard veneer preparation. These teeth would have to be prepared taking into account changing the facial contours, moving the major and minor embrasures, and altering the interproximal contact length. To visualize these changes and determine the preparation necessary, it is advisable to use a study model that can be prepared as if working on patients. The model provides the opportunity to reversibly modify the periodontal

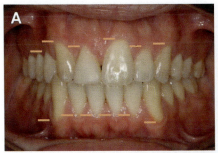
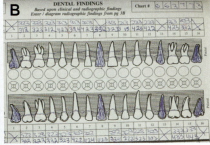

Fig. 3. (A) Discrepancy in gingival height and architecture of the gingival zenith adds to the lack of cosmetic appearance and shows the alterations needed. (B) Perio charting makes clear that the desired alterations to the soft tissue would invade biological width and require osseous recontouring.

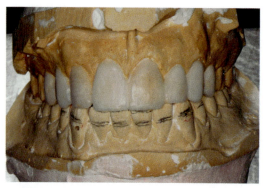

Fig. 4. Wax up showing the desired alterations and indicating the areas of further tooth reduction needed on No. 6 and No. 9.

structures as well as the teeth to arrive at a comprehensive restorative plan. Waxing up the final restorations on the prepared model also reveals the areas where more aggressive tooth preparation is required (**Fig. 4**).

TREATMENT SEQUENCE

The esthetic wax up was duplicated and the resulting model used to make a surgical guide by a suck-down technique with clear matrix material. This clear shell was contoured to the new free gingival margin, but alternatively the matrix can be marked with an indelible pen at this area to serve as a surgical guide. Additional reaction silicone putty was used on the model to create an incisal preparation guide and a matrix for the temporary veneers.

The gingival zeniths of the teeth in the position of No. 5 to No. 8 were altered in both height and shape to conform to the contralateral side using a diode laser (**Fig. 5**). The resulting gingiva was probed to determine any areas where the biological width had been violated as indicated by a lack of periodontal pocket. Wherever this evaluation indicated the need to reestablish the biological width, an erbium:YAG laser was used to perform flapless osteoplasty to move the osseous crest 3 mm from the new free gingival margin (**Fig. 6**). Because the erbium laser is end cutting only, it can be used with a flapless technique to cut through the connective tissue attachment and raise the osseous crest. The erbium laser has been shown to cut bone comparatively

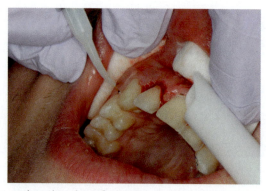

Fig. 5. Diode laser used to alter the soft tissue to the desired height and contour independent of considerations of biological width.

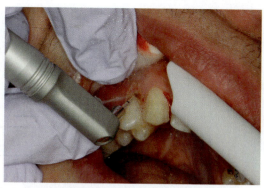

Fig. 6. An erbium laser used in a flapless technique to raise and recontour the osseous crest. The methodology has been shown to be effective in altering osseous structures and safe for root surface.

with a rotary instrument in efficiency and lack of damage to collateral tissues.[2,3] This flapless technique should only be used when there is no need to reduce the horizontal bone width because access would not be possible for facial contouring with an end-cutting instrument. It is essential that the final osseous contour be free of shelves and divots to provide support for the healthy gingival structures. The laser tip was placed subgingivally, axial to the root structure, and worked around the facial tooth attachment with the tip moving apically in a chisel-like motion (see **Fig. 6**). Concerns are often expressed about the effect on the root structure when exposed to the erbium laser. At the settings used for the osseous modification, the erbium laser has been shown to be safe for the root structures and actually provides a better surface for fibroblastic reattachment than scaling and root planing.[4]

Using the laser for the periodontal modification provides the advantage of a predictable result unencumbered by sutures or bleeding. Even with osseous modification, there is little to no postoperative recession. After the periodontal surgery was complete, the teeth were prepared by first altering the facial contours and then breaking contact where required to change the final embrasures and contact length on the teeth in the position of No. 5 to No. 8. This initial step provides a uniform canvas for all of the teeth to be restored. Teeth No. 4 through No. 13 were then prepared for feldspathic porcelain veneers guided by the incisal guide created on the wax up. Adequate reduction was ascertained using the clear matrix created for the surgical guide. A putty matrix of the esthetic wax up was used with Luxatemp (DMG America, Englewood, NJ) to produce temporary veneers (**Fig. 7**). As a final step, a maxillary frenectomy was performed using the diode laser. This procedure was left until the end of the visit to avoid excessive manipulation of the tissues during the restorative procedures.

The patient was seen 2 weeks after the preparation appointment to evaluate the esthetics of the temporary restorations and the tissue response to the periodontal modification. The patient's opinion of the temporaries was discussed, including the form and color, to insure his satisfaction with the final results. A model and photographs of the temporaries including midline and occlusal plane registration was taken to provide the ceramist's laboratory a template for the final veneers. The temporary restorations were removed and the periodontal tissues evaluated. Excellent healing was observed with no inflammation or bleeding, and there was no recession of the free gingival margins beyond the previous preparations (**Fig. 8**). A final poly vinyl siloxane (PVS) impression and bite registration was taken and new temporary veneers created to copy the initial temporaries.

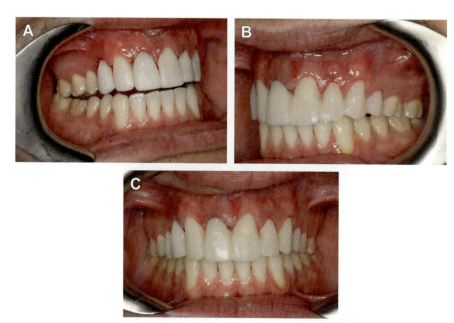

Fig. 7. (A–C) Teeth are prepared for veneers and temporary restorations based on the wax up in place showing changed tooth morphology and altered height and shape of the surrounding structures.

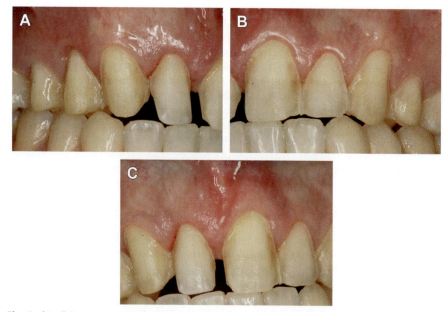

Fig. 8. (A–C) Temporary restorations removed 2 weeks after laser surgery showing healthy tissue with no inflammation or recession.

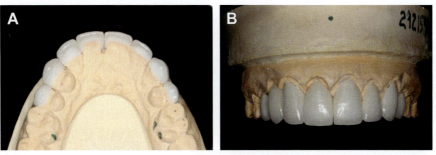

Fig. 9. (*A, B*) Feldspathic porcelain veneers created based on the initial wax up to provide the appropriate tooth morphology and widened and symmetric arch form.

Using the model and photographs of the temporary veneers, the ceramist's laboratory created feldspathic porcelain veneers of the same shape and comparable shade (**Fig. 9**).

The patient returned 2 weeks later, and laboratory-fabricated porcelain veneers (Americus Dental Laboratory) were bonded using a light-cured bonding agent and composite with standard isolation protocol. The dramatic change in tooth morphology and gingival structures is easily seen. Note the gingival health and lack of inflammation or recession indicating the successful restoration of biological width (**Fig. 10**).

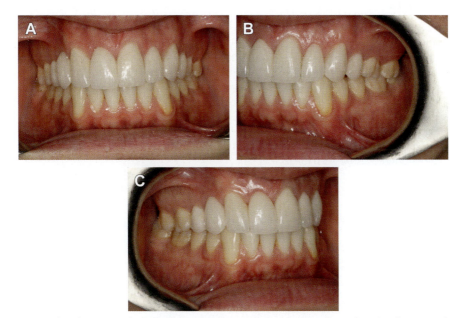

Fig. 10. (*A–C*) Retracted view of the final veneers bonded in place showing harmony in teeth and surrounding structures.

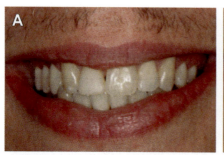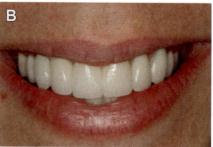

Fig. 11. (A, B) Before and after images clearly show the improvement in esthetics of the smile.

SUMMARY

For patients with a congenitally missing central incisor, there are several options, including implant replacement, full-coverage fixed partial restoration, bonded Maryland bridge, removable prosthetics, or orthodontic repositioning. Although the last treatment is often chosen for congenitally missing lateral incisors, using this method to replace a single central incisor resulted in a particularly unaesthetic result. In this case, modifying the surrounding tissues with 2 different laser wavelengths and creatively prepared and designed porcelain veneers resulted in an attractive smile, harmonious in color and shape. The changes in the overall esthetics and periodontal contours are evident in the before and after images (**Fig. 11**).

For a young man with aspirations in entertainment, this was a result that was personally and professionally significant.

REFERENCES

1. Lewandrowski KU, Lorente C, Schomacker TJ, et al. Use of the Er:AYAG laser for improved plating in maxillofacial surgery: comparison of bone healing in laser and drill osteotomies. Lasers Surg Med 1996;19(1):40–5.
2. Magid K. Effect of cutting speed on collateral thermal damage with a diode laser at 7W CW. Note zone of coagulation increasing as time on tissue increases. Courtesy of research done with Dental Photonics, Walpole MA. Presentation at Academy of Laser Dentistry. Miami FL, 2010.
3. Sasaki KM, Aoki A, Ichinose S, et al. Scanning electron microscopy and FTIR spectroscopy analysis of bone removal using Er:YAG and CO2 lasers. J Periodontol 2002;73:643–52.
4. Moritz W, Kluger U. Changes in root surface morphology and fibroblast adherence after Er:YAG laser irradiation. J Oral Laser Appl 2002;2:83–93.

Simple Case Treatment Planning: Diastema Closure

Vincent Calamia, DDS*, Alexandria Pantzis, DDS

KEYWORDS

- Diastema • Veneers • Smile evaluation form • Laser

KEY POINTS

- This article demonstrates the use of a smile evaluation form as an adjunct in arriving at a diagnosis and developing a treatment plan for a patient desiring Diastema closure.
- It also shows the importance of the diagnostic wax-up for temporization and visualization of case outcome.
- The case also demonstrates the use of soft tissue lasers to create a gingival harmony that enhanced the resulting esthetics.
- Feldspathic porcelain was used for the final restorations because they provide optimal esthetics and translucency.

The patient, a young woman in her early twenties, presented to the Honors Esthetics Clinic at New York University (NYU) College of Dentistry. Her chief complaint was the large diastema between teeth numbers 8 and 9 (**Fig. 1**). Possible causes of the diastema were evaluated and found to be the impact of the low maxillary frenum and possibly an anterior tongue thrust. To completely evaluate the patient, an American Academy of Cosmetic Dentistry series of photographs were taken (**Fig. 2**), a periodontal evaluation performed, and diagnostic casts made. An NYU College of Dentistry Smile Evaluation Form (SEF) (**Fig. 3**) was completed. Problems identified in the SEF included the following:

- Poor width-to-length ratio of the central incisors (**Fig. 4**)
- Poor gingival zeniths position (very asymmetrical) (**Fig. 5**)
- Poor axial inclination of the anterior teeth (**Fig. 6**)
- Poor anterior proportion of teeth (**Fig. 7**)
- A dental midline, not coincidental with the patient's facial midline (**Fig. 8**).

The authors have nothing to disclose.
Private Practice, New York, NY, USA
* Corresponding author.
E-mail address: vincalamia@gmail.com

Dent Clin N Am 59 (2015) 655–664
http://dx.doi.org/10.1016/j.cden.2015.03.010
0011-8532/15/$ – see front matter © 2015 Elsevier Inc. All rights reserved.

dental.theclinics.com

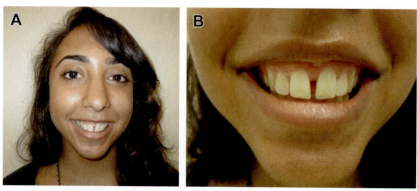

Fig. 1. (*A*) Preoperative facial view. (*B*) Preoperative smile.

The phonetic analysis helped determine the incisal edge position; alginate impressions were taken to initiate a diagnostic wax-up and a matrix was formed to allow an overlay try-in of the planed appearance of the final case (**Fig. 9**).

Analysis of the patient's swallowing pattern was within normal limits and without an anterior tongue thrust. It was determined that the cause of the diastema was a very thick frenum with a "crestal position" (close to the apex of the ridge). Alternative treatments were evaluated and discussed with the patient, including full orthodontic correction, minor tooth movement to space the teeth before restorative changes, which usually results in minimizing restorative tooth reduction and a completely restorative process. The patient declined further orthodontic intervention. She had had previous orthodontic treatment with serial extraction of her first premolars numbers 5, 12, 21, and 28. The patient also decided against composite restorations because of the

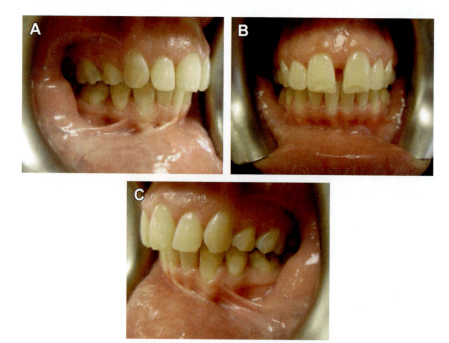

Fig. 2. (*A–C*) Retracted views.

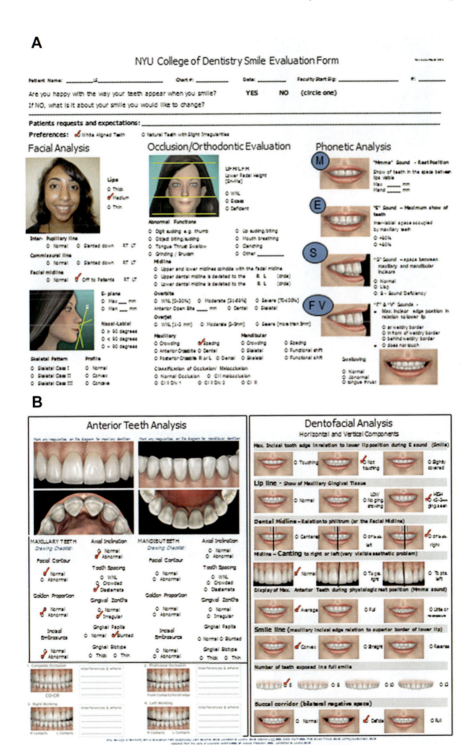

Fig. 3. (*A*) Top of smile evaluation form. (*B*) Anterior teeth and dentofacial analysis on smile evaluation form.

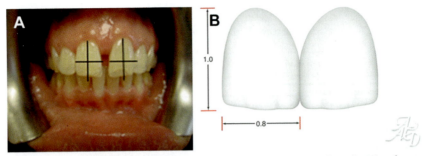

Fig. 4. (*A*) Discrepancy in the width-to-length ratio. (*B*) Ideal width-to-length ratio of central incisors. ([*B*] *Courtesy of* American Academy of Cosmetic Dentistry, Madison, WI; with permission.)

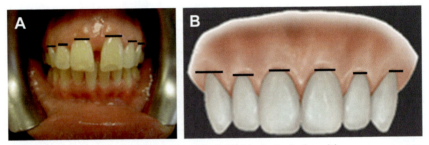

Fig. 5. (*A*) Poor gingival zeniths, asymmetrical. (*B*) Ideal gingival zeniths.

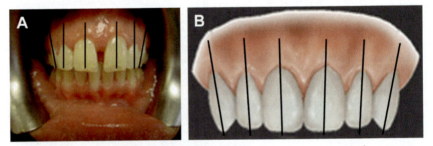

Fig. 6. (*A*) Poor axial inclination. (*B*) Ideal axial inclination, now symmetrical.

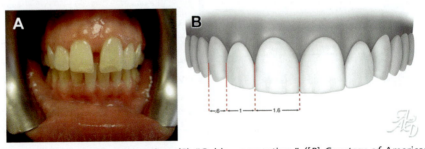

Fig. 7. (*A*) Poor anterior proportion. (*B*) "Golden proportion." ([*B*] *Courtesy of* American Academy of Cosmetic Dentistry, Madison, WI; with permission.)

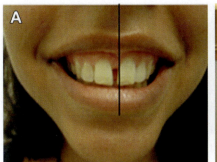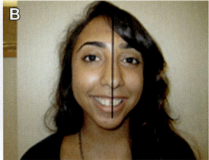

Fig. 8. (*A*) Dental midline is off to the patient's right. (*B*) Obvious discrepancy between facial and dental midlines.

shading, maintenance, and discoloration over time. Porcelain veneers were the restoration chosen by the patient because of their natural esthetic appearance and history of longevity without constant maintenance.

TREATMENT PLAN

The restorative treatment plan included periodontal modification of the gingival architecture, maxillary frenectomy, and feldspathic porcelain veneers from teeth numbers 4 through 13. Modifications of the gingival architecture included movement of the gingival zenith position and eventually providing slightly oversized veneers in the gingival embrasure to allow the gingival papilla between teeth numbers 8 and 9 to go from blunted to more knife-edged. Closing a large diastema has 2 major difficulties. The first challenge is to close the diastema without making the width of the central incisors out of proportion with the length as well as keeping a natural proportion of the width of the central incisors to the widths of the adjacent teeth. The second difficulty in closing a large diastema is avoiding a ledge at the gingival aspect of the contact area that would be a plaque and food trap. This shape would also result in an overly wide base of the papilla, out of harmony with the rest of the arch.

An esthetic wax-up was created to visualize the final result. To determine the ideal width of the central incisors, the "golden percentage" was used.[1] This measurement uses the cuspid-to-cuspid distance visible from the facial view and divides the space into 25% for each central incisor, 15% for the lateral incisor, and 10% for the visible

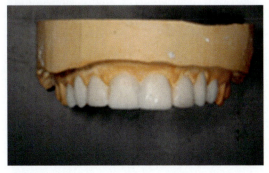

Fig. 9. Diagnostic wax-up.

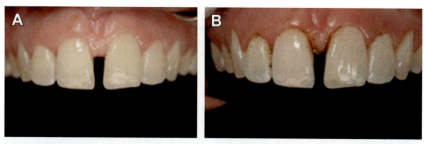

Fig. 10. (*A*) Poor gingival zeniths before laser treatment. (*B*) Soft tissue laser improves the gingival zeniths and mesial gingival of both central incisors.

portion of the cuspid. These measurements are used as a starting point and can be modified based on the curvature of the arch and the reality of the clinical conditions. The wax-up was also used to create an incisal preparation guide and putty matrix for fabrication of the provisionals.

PERIODONTAL CONSIDERATIONS

Dealing with a large maxillary midline diastema presents soft tissue challenges. Because the teeth being treated are "mesialized,"[2] the gingival zeniths of the teeth must also be moved mesially to provide the correct axial inclination of the final restoration. The intrusive maxillary frenum must be removed along with the reticular fibers to avoid reopening of the diastema. To avoid a ledge at the gingival aspect of the contact between the central incisors, the papilla must be narrowed at the base and the troughed to permit the veneer preparation to be started subgingivally and terminate lingually. This design will permit the dental laboratory to create restorations with a proper emergence profile and contours. In numerous cases, one of the authors and supervising faculty have found no significant gingival recession when doing gingivoplasty with a properly controlled diode laser at the same visit as the veneer preparation (**Fig. 10**).

RESTORATIVE CONSIDERATIONS

To close a large diastema while maintaining proper esthetic proportion, it is necessary to "mesialize" the teeth, removing tooth structure from the distal aspects and adding to the mesial surfaces with the porcelain veneers. This reshaping was the first step of the preparation, guided by the incisal preparation guide created on the wax-up. The teeth were then prepared with a standard preparation for feldspathic porcelain veneers (**Fig. 11**). Temporary veneers were fabricated using the

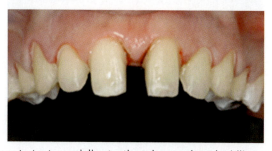

Fig. 11. Preparations to try to mesialize teeth and move dental midline to the patient's left.

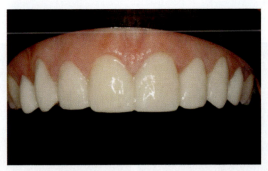

Fig. 12. Provisionals simulating the final result.

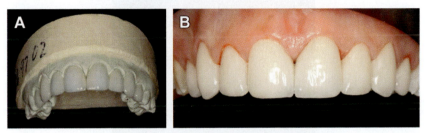

Fig. 13. (*A*) Porcelain veneers on the working model. (*B*) Cemented porcelain veneers day of insertion.

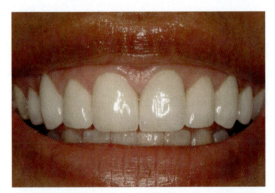

Fig. 14. Two-week recall. Note the gingival papilla between numbers 8 and 9.

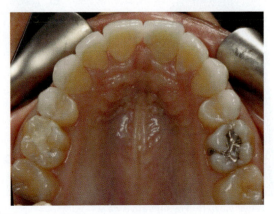

Fig. 15. Incisal view.

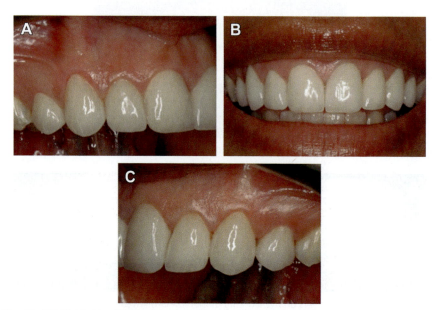

Fig. 16. (*A*) Right side. (*B*) Frontal view. (*C*) Left side.

putty matrix of the wax-up, and Luxatemp provisionals were fabricated to provide an opportunity to evaluate the esthetics and function of the restorative changes (**Fig. 12**).

The patient returned in 2 weeks for evaluation. The tissue frenectomy and surrounding gingival tissue were completely healed. The patient approved the color, shape, and function of the temporaries, final poly-vinyl siloxane impressions (Reprosil Medium body), and bite registration (Reprosil Quixx Putty Heavy body). The new dental midline is determined by transferal of the facial midline onto the final impression tray. The technician can then transfer the location of the new dental midline to his working cast (**Fig. 13**).

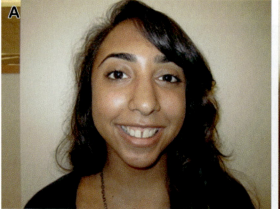
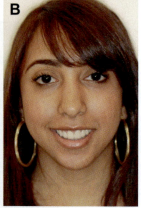

Fig. 17. (*A*) Preoperative view. (*B*) Postoperative view.

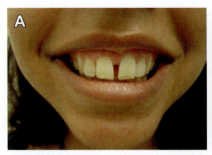 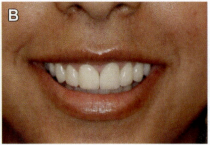

Fig. 18. (*A*) Before photograph. (*B*) After photograph.

The patient returned in 2 weeks, and the final porcelain veneers were bonded using Choice 2 Light Cured Veneer Cement (Bisco, Shaumburg, IL, USA). Occlusion and contacts were checked, and excess cement was removed.

SUMMARY

Closing a large maxillary diastema is a fairly common request of modern-day patients. Although it may seem like a simple, straightforward procedure, it is actually very difficult to accomplish while maintaining proper tooth and interdental proportions, emergence profile, and gingival architecture. The steps presented in this article are those used in the Honors Esthetics Clinic at NYU College of Dentistry and can provide a guide that can result in both a physiologic and an esthetic result (see **Fig. 13**; **Figs. 14–18**).

ACKNOWLEDGMENTS

The authors would also like to offer special thanks to the mentorship of Dr. Kenneth Magid in the Case.

REFERENCES

1. Snow SR. Esthetic smile analysis of maxillary anterior tooth width: the golden percentage. J Esthet Dent 1999;11(4):177–84.
2. Oquendo A, Brea L, David S. Diastema: correction of excessive spaces in the esthetic zone. Dent Clin North Am 2011;55(2):265–81.

FURTHER READINGS

Beasley WK, Maskeroni AJ, Moon MG, et al. The orthodontic and restorative treatment of a large diastema: a case report. Gen Dent 2004;52(1):37–41.
Celenza F. Restorative-orthodontic inter-relations. In: Tarnow D, Chu S, Kim J, editors. Aesthetic restorative dentistry principles and practice. Mahwah (NJ): Montage Media; 2008. p. 427–57.
Chiche G. Proportion, display, and length for successful esthetic planning. In: Cohen M, editor. Interdisciplinary treatment planning. Hanover Park (IL): Quintessence Publishing; 2008. p. 147.
Chu S, Tarnow D, Bloom M. Diagnosis, etiology. In: Tarnow D, Chu S, Kim J, editors. Aesthetic restorative dentistry principles and practice. Mahwah (NJ): Montage Media; 2008. p. 1–25.

Chu S, Tarnow DP, Tan Y, et al. Papilla proportions in the maxillary anterior dentition. Int J Periodontics Restorative Dent 2009;29(4):385–93.

Chu SJ. Range and mean of individual tooth width of the maxillary anterior dentition. Pract Proced Aesthet Dent 2007;19(4):209–15.

Chu SJ, Tan J, Stappert CF, et al. Gingival zenith positions and levels of the maxillary anterior dentition. J Esthet Restor Dent 2009;21(2):113–20.

Dawson PE. The envelope of function. In: Functional occlusion: from TMJ to smile design. St Louis (MO): Mosby Elsevier; 2007. p. 141–7.

De Araujo EM Jr, Fortkamp S, Baratieri LN. Closure of diastema and gingival recontouring using direct adhesive restorations: a case report. J Esthet Restor Dent 2009;21(4):229–40.

Furuse AY, Franco EJ, Mondelli J. Esthetic and functional restoration for an anterior open occlusal relationship with multiple diastemata: a multidisciplinary approach. J Prosthet Dent 2008;99(2):91–4.

Furuse AY, Herkrath FJ, Franco EJ, et al. Multidisciplinary management of anterior diastemata: clinical procedures. Pract Proced Aesthet Dent 2007;19(3): 185–91.

Gracis S, Chu S. The anterior and posterior determinants of occlusion and their relationship to the aesthetic restorative dentistry principles and practice. Mahwah (NJ): Montage Media; 2008. p. 65–97.

Gurel G, Chu S, Kim J. Restorative space management. In: Tarnow D, Chu S, Kim J, editors. Aesthetic restorative dentistry practice principles and practice. Mahwah (NJ): Montage Media; 2008. p. 405–25.

Gurel G. Porcelain laminate veneers for diastema closure. In: The science and art of PLV. Ergolding (Germany): Quintessence Publishing; 2003. p. 369–92.

Sarver DM. Principles of cosmetic dentistry in orthodontics: part 1. Shape and proportionality of anterior teeth. Am J Orthod Dentofacial Orthop 2004;126(6): 749–53.

Sulikowski A. Essential in aesthetics. In: Tarnow D, Chu S, Kim J, editors. Aesthetic restorative dentistry principles and practice. Mahwah (NJ): Montage Media; 2008. p. 27–63.

Tarnow D, Cho SC. The interdental papillae. In: Tarnow D, Chu S, Kim J, editors. Aesthetic restorative dentistry principles and practice. Mahwah (NJ): Montage Media; 2008. p. 367–81.

Tarnow DP, Magner AW, Fletcher P. The effect of the distance from the contact point to the crest of the bone on the presence or absence of the interproximal dental papilla. J Periodontol 1992;63:995–6.

Waldman AB. Smile design for the adolescent patient-interdisciplinary management of anterior tooth size discrepancies. J Calif Dent Assoc 2008;36(5): 365–72.

Ward DH. Proportional smile design using the RED proportion. Dent Clin North Am 2001;45(1):143–54.

Management of an Adult with Class III Malocclusion, Gummy Smile, and Spaced Dentition

 CrossMark

Sameera Babar, DDS[a], John R. Calamia, DMD[b],*,
Jerry M. Sorrel, DDS[c]

KEYWORDS

• Class III malocclusion • Multidiscipline • Aesthetics

KEY POINTS

• This case report presents an interdisciplinary approach to achieve an aesthetically pleasing smile with a functioning occlusion in a patient with a class III malocclusion and a maxillary tooth/jaw size discrepancy.

• Using such adjuncts to treatment planning as a smile evaluation form, radiographs, and initial study casts, a plan for multidiscipline treatment was designed, sequenced, and carried through so that the final treatment objectives were realized with good aesthetics and a functional occlusion.

• Minimal Orthodontic movement was provided to allow equal distribution of space allowing conservative preparation for eventual restorations and Laser removal of excessive soft tissue addresses gummy smile.

PATIENT BACKGROUND AND CHIEF CONCERNS

The patient is a 27 year old African American man (**Figs. 1** and **2**) and is a self-described actor/model. He presented to New York University College of Dentistry (NYUCD) for dental evaluation to improve his smile and facial appearance (see **Figs. 1** and **2**).

Medical history had no significant findings, no allergies reported, and no current medications.

Blood pressure was 110/70. Pulse was 71 beats per minute, and respiration was 19 breaths per minute. Weight was 200 lbs, and height was 6' 1''. Body mass index was 24.6.

The authors have nothing to disclose.
[a] Peninsula Dental center, 1101 Healthway Dr, Salisbury, MD 21804, USA; [b] Department of Cariology and Comprehensive Care, New York University, College of Dentistry, NY 10010, USA; [c] Department of Orthodontics, New York University, College of Dentistry, NY 10010, USA
* Corresponding author.
E-mail address: jrc1@nyu.edu

Dent Clin N Am 59 (2015) 665–674
http://dx.doi.org/10.1016/j.cden.2015.03.002
0011-8532/15/$ – see front matter © 2015 Elsevier Inc. All rights reserved.

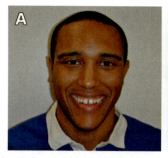
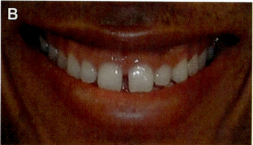

Fig. 1. (*A, B*) Patient at initial evaluation.

DENTAL HISTORY

Regular dental care reports indicated "dark teeth, large spaces, too much gum showing."

The patient had a class III malocclusion with a class III skeletal pattern. A smile evaluation form (**Fig. 2**) and other treatment planning adjuncts (**Figs. 3–7**) were performed to help formulate what specialty disciplines would be involved in the case work-up.

The panoramic radiograph revealed missing teeth #1, #16, #17, #32, and root canal therapy (RCT) and crowns on teeth #15 and #19. Composite fillings could be found on teeth #2, #3, #4, #5, #12, #13, and #14 in the maxilla and teeth #18, #20, #29, #30, and #31 in the mandible. There was no evidence of condylar pathology.

Occlusal photographs were taken of the maxillary and mandibular views, and along with the diagnostic casts, spacing/crowding was measured (**Figs. 5** and **6**).

PRIMARY OBJECTIVES

After reviewing the treatment plan adjuncts, it was obvious that a multidisciplinary approach to treatment was needed.

The restorative dentist invited the orthodontist and the periodontist for a sit-down discussion of the case to formulate not only a formal treatment plan but also a sequence of treatment for this case.

The comprehensive orthodontic treatment objective was to improve the patient's facial profile, achieve adequate overjet and overbite, and provide space distribution among maxillary anterior teeth as well as a harmonious and stable occlusal relationship.

The periodontal treatment objective was to maintain a healthy gingival foundation and to provide minor gingivoplasty to achieve ideal gingival zeniths and an overall aesthetic gingival display. The restorative treatment objective was to meet the patient's initial concerns of spacing and gingival gummy appearance while providing aesthetically pleasing smile and improving the total facial appearance of the patient.

The following sequence of treatment was discussed and would be presented to the patient at the next visit.

Phase I: This phase consists of operative caries control and hygiene instruction.

Phase II: This phase consists of comprehensive orthodontic treatment.

Phase III: This phase consists of perio-treatment to address crown lengthening and gingival zenith design.

Phase IV: A postorthodontic SEF would be performed and a second restorative consultation done. New Impressions of the current occlusion would be taken and new diagnostic casts created. A retainer would be made to assure no movement of the teeth while restorative work is designed and finished. A diagnostic

A

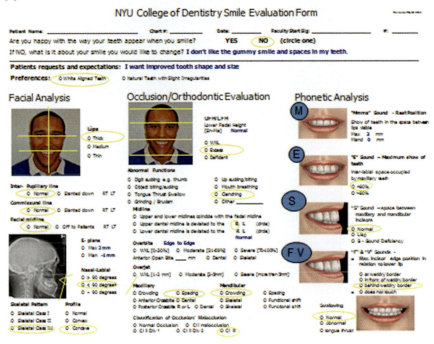

B

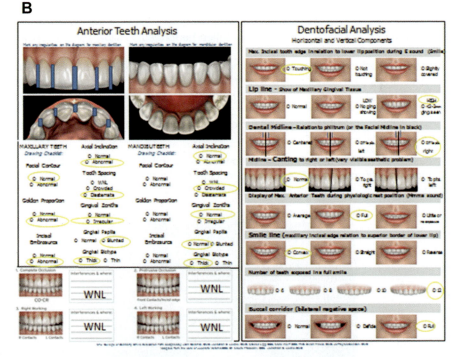

Fig. 2. (*A*, *B*) New York University College of Dentistry smile evaluation form.

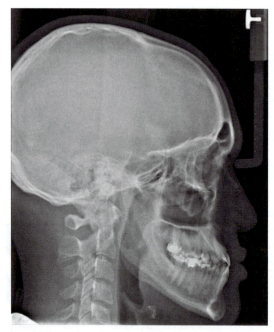

Fig. 3. Right lateral cephalometric radiograph. This view reveals a normo-divergent, class III skeletal pattern with an average lower facial height, average facial convexity, and slightly acute nasolabial angle.

wax-up would be done, providing a 3-dimensional version of the expected final restorations positions. Matrices would then be formed to allow for provisionals to be made for try-in.

Phase V: Restorative preparations, impressioning, laboratory fabrication, try-in, placement, and finishing are accomplished. Postrestorative appointments to finalize occlusal adjustments would be needed. Fabrication of protective night guard would be required.

Phase VI: Scheduled recalls every 6 months monitoring home care would also be discussed.

Phase I operative and hygiene instruction includes tooth # 18 mesial-occlusal (MO) composite restoration, tooth # 29 distal-occlusal (DO) composite restoration, and tooth # 31 Mesial, Occlusal, and Distal surfaces (MOD) composite restoration.

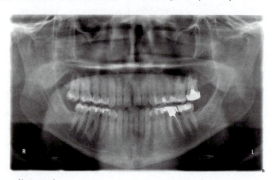

Fig. 4. Panoramic radiograph.

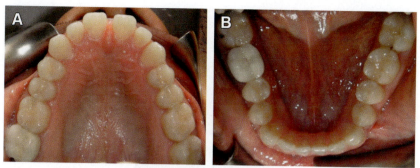

Fig. 5. (*A*) Maxillary arch (spacing = 7 mm). (*B*) Mandibular arch (crowding = 1 mm).

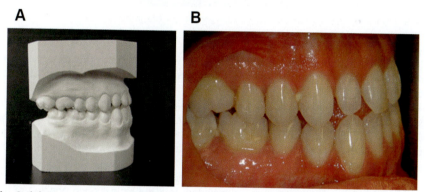

Fig. 6. (*A*) Diagnostic study casts and right side lateral photographs (*B*) revealed a class III molar relationship, class III right canine with teeth #1 and #32 missing.

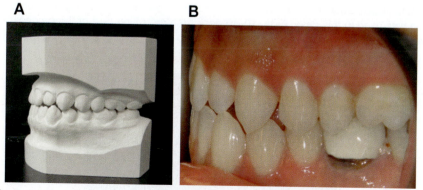

Fig. 7. (*A*) The same diagnostic study casts and left side lateral. (*B*) Photographs revealed a class III molar relationship, and a class 1 canine relationship.

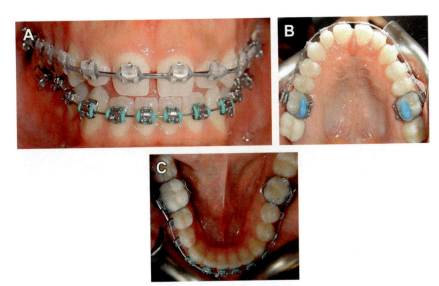

Fig. 8. (*A*) Fixed wire appliances. (*B*) Maxillary view. (*C*) Mandibular view.

In phase II, orthodontic fixed wire appliances were placed to retro-cline the lower anteriors and realign the maxillary teeth to allow equal distribution of spaces to be closed (**Fig. 8**).

In phase III, upon completion of the orthodontic stage, the periodontist may use a blade or a soft tissue laser to remove excess soft tissue to allow a less gummy smile. Biological width must be maintained. In some cases of a high lip line and a very gummy appearance, osseous reduction might be necessary. In this particular case, only a soft tissue laser reduction was necessary (**Fig. 9**).

In phase V, after orthodontics and periodontics are complete, diagnostic casts are again made and a diagnostic wax-up provided. In it the incisal edge position of the maxillary anterior teeth is determined, and space distribution can be addressed using the golden proportion, the golden percentage, or the red proportion, depending upon one's philosophy of anterior aesthetics. The golden proportion is the apparent ratio in size of the central incisor, lateral incisor, and canine, when viewed directly from the front of the patient, so that the central appears 1.6, the lateral appears 1.0 and the canine appears 0.6 in surface visibility in relation to one another. The golden proportion was used in this case. **Figs. 10–16** depict the remaining part of the process, as well as the end results.

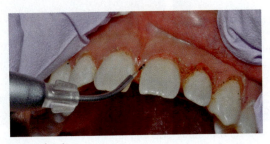

Fig. 9. Soft tissue laser reduction.

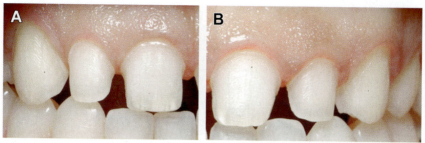

Fig. 10. (*A*) Preparation upper right quadrant. (*B*) Preparation upper left quadrant.

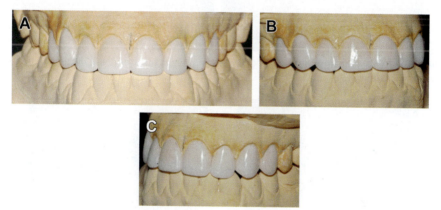

Fig. 11. (*A*) Diagnostic wax-up. (*B*) Wax-up right lateral view. (*C*) Wax-up left lateral view.

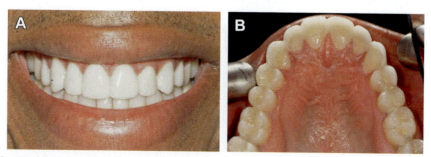

Fig. 12. (*A, B*) Provisionals in place.

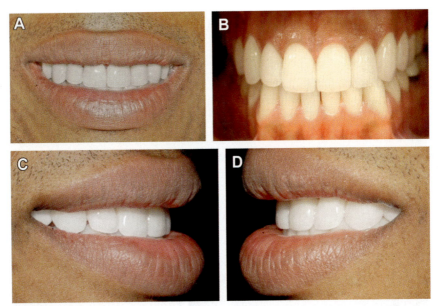

Fig. 13. (*A, B*) Final restorations. (*C*) Right side permanent restorations. (*D*) Left side permanent restorations.

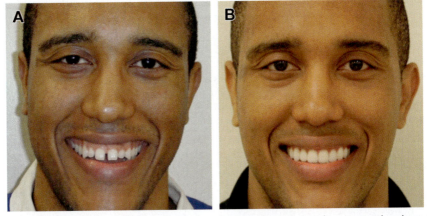

Fig. 14. (*A, B*) Provides a full face comparison of the preoperative and postoperative views of the patient. Note how much more confident and relaxed the post-operative photo appears.

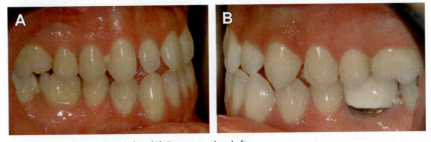

Fig. 15. (*A*) Preoperative right. (*B*) Preoperative left.

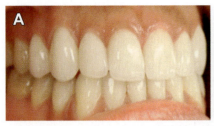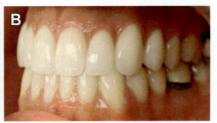

Fig. 16. (*A*) Postoperative right. (*B*) Postoperative left.

Phase VI consists of maintenance and recall:

- Final orthodontic retainer to prevent relapse
- Regular recalls to evaluate caries risk and margin integrity of restorations every 6 months

SUMMARY

In this case, it has been demonstrated that using adjunct guides to treatment planning such as smile evaluation forms, radiographs (full mouth series [FMS], panoramic, cephalometric where needed), and diagnostic casts provides a great understanding of what disciplines will be needed to properly treat the case. The restorative dentist should take the lead and have in mind not only a functional result but an aesthetic success. A sit down or conference should then be organized so that all the health care providers understand their roles in the process and will come to agreement upon the proper sequencing of that care. A team effort to address all the patient's needs can be discussed and can then be conveyed to the patient so that he or she is properly informed as to what is the best course of treatment.

FURTHER READINGS

Beasley WK, Maskeroni AJ, Moon MG, et al. The orthodontic and restorative treatment of a large diastema: a case report. Gen Dent 2004;52(1):37–41.

Calamia JR. Etched porcelain veneer restorations: a twenty year retrospective, vol. II. Montage Media; 2005. American Academy of Cosmetic Dentistry Monograph.

Calamia JR, Calamia CS. Porcelain laminate veneers: reasons for 25 years of success. Dent Clin North Am 2007;51(2):399–417.

Calamia JR, Calamia CS, Magid K, et al. Successful esthetics and cosmetic dentistry for the modern dental practice. Dent Clin North Am 2007;51(2):281–572.

Calamia JR, Calamia CS, Magid K, et al. A multidisciplinary approach to the indirect esthetic treatment of diastemata. Functional Esthetics and Restorative Dentistry. Aegis Communications; 2007.

Calamia JR, Wolff M, Trushkowsky R. Esthetic and cosmetic dentistry for modern dental practice: update 2011. Dent Clin North Am 2011.

Celenza F. Restorative-orthodontic inter-relations. In: Tarnow D, Chu S, Kim J, editors. Aesthetic restorative dentistry principles and practice. Mahwah (NJ): Montage Media; 2008. p. 427–57.

Chiche G. Proportion, display, and length for successful esthetic planning. In: Cohen M, editor. Interdisciplinary treatment planning. Hanover Park (IL): Quintessence Publishing; 2008. p. 147.

Chu SJ. Range and mean of individual tooth width of the maxillary anterior dentition. Pract Proced Aesthet Dent 2007;19(4):209–15.

Chu S, Tarnow D, Bloom M. Diagnosis, etiology. In: Tarnow D, Chu S, Kim J, editors. Aesthetic restorative dentistry principles and practice. Mahwah (NJ): Montage Media; 2008. p. 1–25.

Chu SJ, Tan J, Stappert CF, et al. Gingival zenith positions and levels of the maxillary anterior dentition. J Esthet Restor Dent 2009;21(2):113–20.

Chu S, Tarnow DP, Tan Y, et al. Papilla proportions in the maxillary anterior dentition. Int J Periodontics Restorative Dent 2009;4:385–93.

Dawson P. The envelope of function. In: Functional occlusion: from TMJ to smile design. St Louis (MO): Mosby Elsevier; 2007. p. 141–7.

De Araujo EM Jr, Fortkamp S, Baratieri LN. Closure of diastema and gingival recontouring using direct adhesive restorations, a case report. J Esthet Restor Dent 2009;21(4):229–40.

Furuse AY, Herkrath FJ, Franco EJ, et al. Multidisciplinary management of anterior Diastemata: clinical procedures. Pract Proced Aesthet Dent 2007;19(3):185–91.

Furuse AY, Franco EJ, Mondelli J. Esthetic and functional restoration for an anterior open occlusal relationship with multiple Diastemata: a multidisciplinary approach. J Prosthet Dent 2008;99(2):91–4.

Gracis S, Chu S. The anterior and posterior determinants of occlusion and their relationship to the aesthetic restorative dentistry principles and practice. Mahwah (NJ): Montage Media; 2008. p. 65–97.

Gurel G. Porcelain laminate veneers for diastema closure. In: The science and art of PLV. Ergolding (Germany): Quintessence Publishing; 2003. p. 369–92.

Gurel G, Chu S, Kim J. Restorative space management. In: Tarnow D, Chu S, Kim J, editors. Aesthetic restorative dentistry practice principles and practice. Mahwah (NJ): Montage Media; 2008. p. 405–25.

Sarver DM. Principles of cosmetic dentistry in orthodontics: part 1. Shape and proportionality of anterior teeth. Am J Orthod Dentofacial Orthop 2004;126(6):749–53.

Sulikowski A. Essential in aesthetics. In: Tarnow D, Chu S, Kim J, editors. Aesthetic restorative dentistry principles and practice. Mahwah (NJ): Montage Media; 2008. p. 27–63.

Tarnow DP, Magner AW, Fletcher P. The effect of the distance from the contact point to the crest of the bone on the presence or absence of the interproximal dental papilla. J Periodontol 1992;63:995–6.

Tarnow D, Cho SC. The interdental papillae. In: Tarnow D, Chu S, Kim J, editors. Aesthetic restorative dentistry principles and practice. Mahwah (NJ): Montage Media; 2008. p. 367–81.

Waldman AB. Smile design for the adolescent patient—interdisciplinary management of anterior tooth size discrepancies. J Calif Dent Assoc 2008;36(5):365–72.

Ward DH. Proportional smile design using the RED proportion. Dent Clin North Am 2001;45(1):143–54.

Esthetic Smile Design
Limited Orthodontic Therapy to Position Teeth for Minimally Invasive Veneer Preparation

 CrossMark

Andi-Jean Miro, DDS[a],*, Alex Shalman, DDS[a],
Ramiro Morales, DMD[b], Nicholas J. Giannuzzi, DDS[c,d]

KEYWORDS

- Smile evaluation • Multidisciplined treatment • Diagnostic wax-up
- Porcelain veneers

KEY POINTS

- At present, the standards of dentistry are being elevated, because a greater emphasis is being placed on esthetics along with functionality.
- Minimally invasive dentistry has become an essential component in creating restorations that are both functional and have increased longevity.
- In the following case, the patient underwent 9 months of orthodontic therapy to correct her improper overbite, overjet, and spacing of her dentition to position the teeth for future restorations that were minimally invasive.
- Orthodontic therapy was paramount in positioning the teeth so that the future restorations would have ideal axial inclinations and limit tooth reduction in order to be as minimally invasive as possible.

INTRODUCTION

In the following case, a comprehensive treatment plan was created to address the chief concerns of the patient. The initial treatment plan was completed with the use of the Smile Evaluation Form (**Fig. 1**).[1] To achieve the desired esthetic results, a combination of dental modalities was deemed necessary and included orthodontics as

The authors have nothing to disclose.
[a] Aesthetic Honors Program, Department of Cariology and Comprehensive Care, New York University College of Dentistry, 345 E 24th St, New York, NY 10010, USA; [b] Orthodontics Program, New York University College of Dentistry, 345 E 24th St, New York, NY 10010, USA; [c] Aesthetic Honors Program, Department of Cariology and Comprehensive Care, New York University College of Dentistry, 345 E 24th St, New York, NY 10010, USA; [d] Private Practice, 10 Hunter Ave, Miller Place, NY 11764, USA
* Corresponding author.
E-mail address: andijeanmiro@gmail.com

Dent Clin N Am 59 (2015) 675–687
http://dx.doi.org/10.1016/j.cden.2015.04.001
0011-8532/15/$ – see front matter © 2015 Elsevier Inc. All rights reserved.

dental.theclinics.com

A

NYU College of Dentistry Smile Evaluation Form

Released JIRC Aug 2014

| Patient Name: | | Chart #: | | Date: | | Faculty Start Sig: | | #: |

Are you happy with the way your teeth appear when you smile?   YES   NO   (circle one)

If NO, what is it about your smile you would like to change?

Patients requests and expectations:

Preferences: O White Aligned Teeth   O Natural Teeth with Slight Irregularities

Facial Analysis

Inter- Pupillary line
O Normal   O Slanted down   RT LT

Commissural line
O Normal   O Slanted down   RT LT

Facial midline
O Normal   O Off to Patients   RT LT

E- plane
O Max _____ mm
O Man _____ mm

Nasal-Labial
O > 90 degrees
O < 90 degrees
O = 90 degrees

Lips
O Thick
O Medium
O Thin

Skeletal Pattern
O Skeletal Class I
O Skeletal Class II
O Skeletal Class III

Profile
O Normal
O Convex
O Concave

Occlusion/Orthodontic Evaluation

UFH/LFH
Lower Facial Height
[Sn-Me]
O WNL
O Excess
O Deficient

Abnormal Functions
O Digit sucking e.g. thumb
O Object biting/sucking
O Tongue Thrust Swallow
O Grinding / Bruxism
O Lip sucking/biting
O Mouth breathing
O Clenching
O Other _____

Midline
O Upper and lower midlines coincide with the facial midline
O Upper dental midline is deviated to the   R   L   (circle)
O Lower dental midline is deviated to the   R   L   (circle)

Overbite
O WNL [0-30%]   O Moderate [31-69%]   O Severe [70-100%]
Anterior Open Bite _____ mm   O Dental   O Skeletal

Overjet
O WNL [1-2 mm]   O Moderate [3-5mm]   O Severe [more than 5mm]

Maxillary
O Crowding   O Spacing
O Dental
O Anterior Crossbite   O Dental
O Posterior Crossbite R or L   O Dental

Mandibular
O Crowding   O Spacing
O Skeletal   O Functional shift
O Skeletal
O Skeletal   O Functional shift

Classification of Occlusion/ Malocclusion
O Normal Occlusion   O Cl I malocclusion
O Cl II Div 1   O Cl II Div 2   O Cl

Phonetic Analysis

M

"M" Sound - Rest Position
Show of teeth in the space
between lips visible
Max _____ mm
Mand _____ mm

E

"E" Sound – Maximum show of teeth
Interlabial space occupied
by maxillary teeth
O <80%
O >80%

S

"S" Sound – space between maxillary and mandibular incisors
O Normal
O Lisp
O S - Sound Deficiency

FV

"F" & "V" Sounds -
O Max. Incisor edge position in relation to lower lip
O at wet/dry border
O in front of wet/dry border
O behind wet/dry border

Swallowing
O Normal
O Abnormal
O tongue thrust

Fig. 1. (A) Smile Evaluation Form, page 1. (B) Smile Evaluation Form, page 2. (*Courtesy of* John Calamia, DMD; Mitchell Lipp, DDS; and Jonathan B. Levine, DMD, GoSMILE Aesthetics, 923 5th Avenue, New York, NY 10021; *Adapted from* Leonard Abrams, 255 South Seventeenth Street, Philadelphia, PA 19103, 1987; and Dr Mauro Fradeani, Esthetic Rehabilitation in Fixed Prosthodontics Quintessence Publishing Co, Inc, Carol Stream, IL, 2004.)

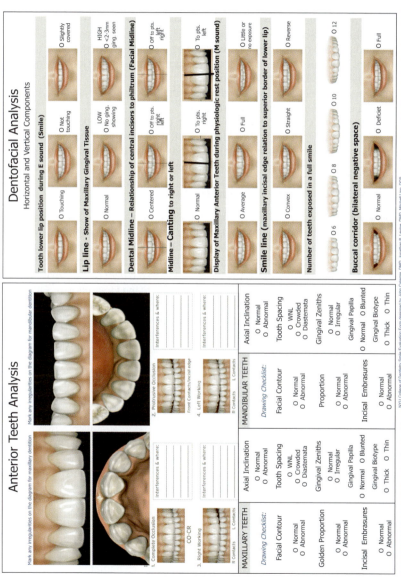

Fig. 1. (*continued*)

well as restorative therapy. After completing the orthodontic treatment, a new Smile Evaluation Form[1] was administered in order to help determine the appropriate final treatment plan. The final restorations were placed, and a retention plan was implemented so that the restorations would be maintained over time.

PATIENT BACKGROUND AND CHIEF CONCERN

The patient presented to the New York University College of Dentistry (NYUCD) Undergraduate Clinic. After the new patient intake protocol was completed, it was determined that the patient's chief concern was the esthetic appearance of her smile. At this point, she was referred from the Undergraduate General Dentistry group to the Honors in Aesthetic Dentistry Program.

At the beginning of her esthetic evaluation, the patient stated "I would like to close the spaces on the top and improve my smile."

Using the NYUCD Smile Evaluation Form,[1] in addition to radiographs, photographs, and mounted study casts, it was determined that the most conservative way to achieve the maximum esthetic result would be to treat this case with a combination of orthodontic and restorative treatment modalities.

SMILE EVALUATION FORM: FACIAL ANALYSIS

The patient presented with a normal horizontal interpupillary line and commissural line (**Fig. 2**). The lower third of her face was slightly larger than the other thirds of her face. She had a slightly asymmetric face with a strong pronounced chin, which was deviated to the left. The patient had an average-sized nose and a thin upper lip.

The patient's maxillary dental midline was 1 mm to the right of the facial midline, and the mandibular dental midline was 1.5 mm to the left of the facial midline. From the profile, her face was slightly concave. When analyzing from the profile in relation to Dr Robert Rickett's esthetic plane,[2] an imaginary line drawn from the tip of the nose to the tip of the chin, her maxillary lip appeared to be 10 mm from the E-plane and her mandibular lip appeared to be 6 mm from the E-plane. Her nasolabial angle appeared obtuse.

SMILE EVALUATION FORM: OCCLUSAL ANALYSIS

The patient's maxillary arch was U shaped and symmetric with 8 mm of spacing. The patient's mandibular arch was also U shaped and symmetric with 4 mm of spacing (**Fig. 3**). The patient denied any parafunctional or dysfunctional habits, but on clinical examination there was evidence of wear on her posterior teeth. It was based on this initial analysis that she was then referred to NYUCD Orthodontic Department for a consultation and comprehensive orthodontic workup.

OTHER DIAGNOSTIC AIDS AND ORTHODONTIC ANALYSIS

The patient presented to the orthodontic clinic and was evaluated using orthodontic parameters including diagnostic photographs, models, and lateral cephalometric and panoramic imaging (**Fig. 4**). The patient had an asymmetric face with her chin deviated to the left, prognathic concave profile, average nose, obtuse nasolabial angle, and thin and competent upper and lower lips, which were behind the E-plane by 10 and 6 mm, respectively. Intraorally, her molar Angle classification was Class I and canine relationship, Class I. Her overbite was 1 mm (10%) with 1 mm of overjet. She had generalized spacing with 8 mm in the maxillary arch and 4 mm in the mandibular.

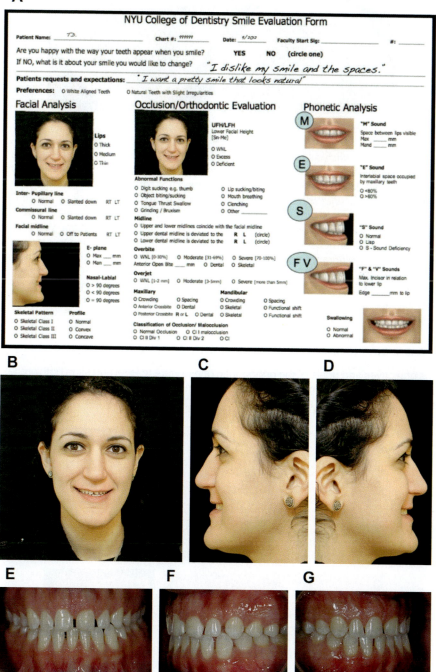

Fig. 2. (*A*) The patient's initial Smile Evaluation Form. (*B*) Initial full face photograph. (*C*) Initial left profile. (*D*) Initial right profile. (*E*) Initial center retracted image. (*F*) Initial left retracted image. (*G*) Initial right retracted image.

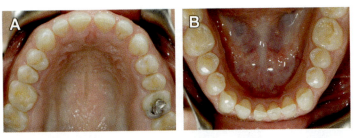

Fig. 3. (*A, B*) Occlusal analysis.

Cephalometric analysis revealed a Class III skeletal pattern with a normodivergent mandibular plane, long mandible and prominent chin, slightly proclined upper incisors, and retroclined lower incisors. A primary consideration for this orthodontic treatment was the shallow overjet and overbite because of her tooth size discrepancy; her maxillary incisors were small and would not benefit from the spaces alone being closed. If these spaces were closed on both the upper and lower arches, the patient would have gone into edge-to-edge incisor relationship or even into an anterior cross-bite because of the difference in tooth size and spacing between the upper and lower arch, as well as her Class III dental tendency and skeletal pattern. The retraction of incisors would have accentuated her concave profile depressing the lower third of her face and accentuating her skeletal Class III skeletal pattern, which would have only worsened with age.

PHASE 1: DIAGNOSIS AND OBJECTIVES OF ORTHODONTIC THERAPY

The objectives and goals of the orthodontic phase were to level and align both arches, maintain molar and canine relationships, distribute the spaces evenly on the maxillary arch, and close the spaces on the mandibular. The goal was to match the maxillary

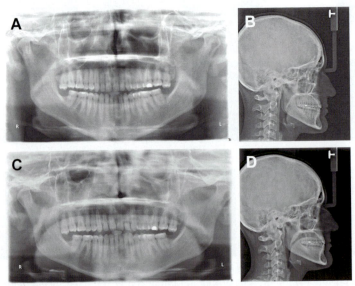

Fig. 4. (*A*) Pan preorthodontic. (*B*) Ceph preorthodontic. (*C*) Pan postorthodontic. (*D*) Ceph postorthodontic.

dental midline to the facial midline and develop adequate overjet and overbite in an ideal position for the veneer preparations.

During the orthodontic consult, the patient was informed that in order to match her maxillary and mandibular dental midlines the treatment duration would be approximately one and a half years. However, the patient wanted to spend the least time in orthodontics and have the most conservative tooth preparation possible, for achieving the best esthetic outcome. As a compromise, the patient understood that postoperatively her maxillary and mandibular dental midlines would not coincide but would be close. According to Kokich and colleagues,[3] most general dentists and lay people when looking at a smile are unable to detect a midline deviation unless it is greater than 4 mm.

Maxillary and mandibular arches were bonded with interactive self-ligating brackets GAC-R (In-Ovation Self Ligating Brackets, Densply) and the spaces were redistributed using NiTi open coil springs (Dentsply, New York, PA).

One of the most important details of an interdisciplinary case is the importance of communication between the orthodontist and the restorative dentist. It is the inclination of the orthodontist to want to close spaces completely, whereas it is the view of the restorative dentist, using a different diagnostic parameter, that spaces should be minimized and distributed equally among teeth to be restored. Throughout the orthodontic treatment, both the orthodontist and Aesthetic Honors Program examined the patient periodically to determine if treatment was progressing accordingly.

Reevaluation Postorthodontics

After approximately 9 months of orthodontic treatment, it was determined that the maxillary and mandibular spacing were ideally situated for restorative treatment to begin (**Fig. 5**). The brackets and arch wire were removed. On completion of orthodontic treatment, the patient was given a maxillary and mandibular Essix retainer (Dentsply) to wear full time until the restorative aspect of treatment could be completed.

Smile Evaluation After Orthodontic Treatment

The patient was reevaluated postorthodontics using the Smile Evaluation Form (**Fig. 6**A).[1] The interpupillary line, commissural line, and facial midline were maintained and were normal.

Postorthodontics (see **Fig. 6**; **Figs. 7** and **8**), the maxillary dental midline coincided with the facial midline. The lower dental midline was 1 mm to the left of the facial midline. The axial inclination of tooth 7 was slightly distally inclined but did not warrant further orthodontic treatment and could be corrected with the final restorations. The gingival zeniths were esthetically ideal.[4] The incisal embrasures were abnormal, and because of the spacing between the teeth, the gingival papillae were blunted.

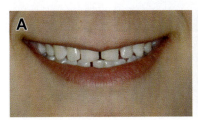 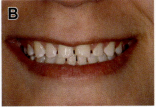

Fig. 5. Orthodontics overview. (*A*) Pretreatment. (*B*) Postorthodontic treatment.

A

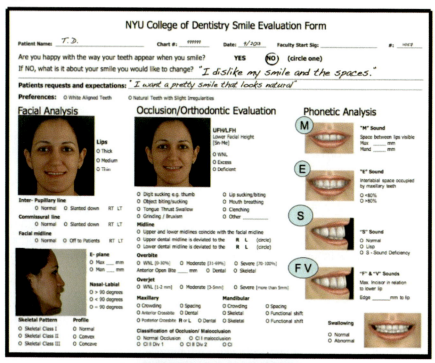

B

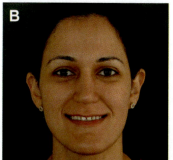

C 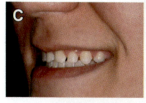   **D** 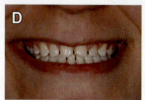   **E**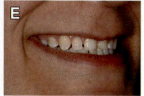

Fig. 6. (*A*) Smile Evaluation Form, page 1, postorthodontics. (*B*) Postorthodontics full face. (*C*) Postorthodontic, nonretracted (*Left*). (*D*) Postorthodontic, nonretracted. (*E*) Postorthodontic, nonretracted (*Right*).

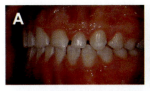 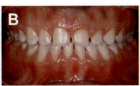 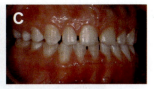

Fig. 7. (*A*) Postorthodontics retracted (*Left*). (*B*) Postorthodontics retracted (*Center*). (*C*) Postorthodontics retracted (*Right*).

The dentofacial analysis evaluated the teeth within the frame of the face and lips. It is important to evaluate facial discrepancies and incorporate them in the evaluation. The patient had a thin upper lip and a reverse low lip line, meaning that in the anterior her lip came down lower than in the posterior. When evaluating the patient's smile, the incisal edges of the maxillary teeth do not touch the lower lip and the position of the teeth in relation to the lower lip are reverse, meaning the incisors were shorter than the posterior teeth. The patient had a full buccal corridor, and when she smiled, she showed back the first molars.

Finalized Treatment Plan

New mounted diagnostic casts were created at the current postorthodontic position, from which a pretherapeutic wax-up was fabricated (**Fig. 9**A). Initially, teeth 4 to 13 were waxed. This wax-up would serve multiple purposes, and it would act as a blueprint for treatment. Putty impressions of this wax-up were fabricated (Reprosil Putty, vinyl polysiloxane impression material, Dentsply) and used to create buccal/incisal reduction guides, as well as a matrix for fabricating provisionals (see **Fig. 9**B).

The patient wanted restorations that would blend and look natural next to her unprepared teeth. This case is an additive case meaning that the final restorations would be adding width and length to existing teeth. Using the matrix of the wax-up the restorations were tried in and evaluated using Luxatemp provisional material (DMG America, Englewood, NJ, USA).

It was determined that achieving the patient's ideal esthetic goals, teeth 7 to 10 and 23 to 26 had to be treated. The final planned restorations would be 8 feldspathic porcelain veneers. Two weeks before preparation, both the maxillary and mandibular arches were bleached (Zoom Whitening [Philips, Andover, MA]) to have a lighter starting shade and overall whiter and brighter end result. After the restorations were inserted, an Essix clear retainer (Dentsply) was used to retain the new orthodontic position as well as the restored dentition after treatment was completed.

Risks were not significant.

The prognosis was excellent.

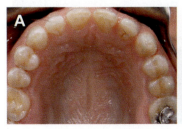 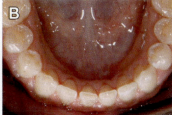

Fig. 8. (*A*) Postorthodontics occlusal (Maxillary). (*B*) Postorthodontics occlusal (Mandibular).

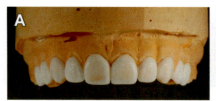
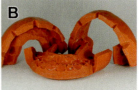

Fig. 9. (*A*) Diagnostic wax-up. (*B*) Matrixes.

PHASE 2: PREPARATION AND PROVISIONALIZATION

It was paramount to the patient that the preparations be as minimally invasive as possible. This fact was taken into consideration in the beginning of the treatment planning process, which was why the patient opted for orthodontic therapy. The preparations were designed to prepare the least amount of tooth structure, to increase longevity,[5] and to take advantage of the strong and predictable porcelain to enamel bond.[6] It is also important to consider that the bond strengths of the resin cement to enamel when the preparations when kept in enamel are significantly higher and more predictable than bond strengths to dentin.[6]

There is much debate when it comes to the idea of prepless veneers versus minimal preparation veneers. Most ceramists prefer a defined and detectable finish line to facilitate the seating of the veneers.[7] In this case, the orthodontic therapy was successful in positioning the teeth so that they required only minimal finishing and placement of a finish line.

In order to be conservative and prepare as little tooth as possible, the esthetic diagnostic wax-up was used. The matrix fabricated from the wax-up was filled with Luxatemp and placed over the teeth much like at the try in appointment (**Fig. 10**B), and this was used as a guide. Teeth 7 to 10 and 23 to 26 were prepared on the facial with 0.5-mm depth cutting bur (Rosenthal-Apa Bur Block 5007901U0, Brasseler [Savannah, GA]) through the provisional (see **Fig. 10**C). The depth cuts were then marked with pencil (see **Fig. 10**D). The facial required no reduction and only the placement of a chamfer finish line. The teeth were prepared as if the provisionals were the actual teeth. A finish line was created as a definitive seat on the facial and was refined with chamfer at the level of the free gingival margin (Two Striper diamond #799, Primer

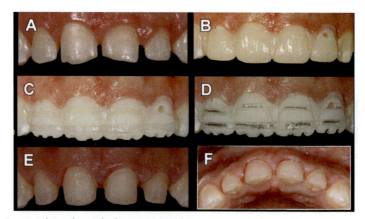

Fig. 10. Preparations through the provisionals.

Dental [Plymouth Meeting, PA]) (see **Fig. 10**E, F). Interproximally, the teeth were not finished with a chamfer finish line but rather prepared straight through, removing any undercut and without a definitive finish line. The incisal edges were rounded off with a soft flex disc (3M ESPE, St. Paul, MN).

The preparations were impressed with medium- and light-body vinyl polysiloxane impression material (Aquasil Ultra, Dentsply). Provisional restorations were fabricated using the putty matrix (Dentsply) from the diagnostic wax-up and using Luxatemp and Luxaflow shade A1 (DMG America). The provisional restorations were considered a test drive for the patient. These provisionals were further adjusted intraorally 24 hours postoperatively to achieve ideal esthetics and occlusion. The provisionals were then impressed and photographed and sent to the laboratory so that the approximate contours could be copied when designing the porcelain restorations (**Fig. 11**).

Laboratory Fabrication

Feldspathic porcelain veneers were selected as the restorative material of choice because it is the most esthetic restorative material and also requires the least amount of tooth reduction.[5]

Eight feldspathic veneers were fabricated on dies that were first overlayed with platinum foil. The veneers were created using different dentin and enamel shades of porcelain (Softspar Creation, Pentron, Orange, CA) to achieve optimal esthetics and matching with the shade of the adjacent teeth. The veneers were glazed, and the platinum foil was removed from the internal surface of the veneers. The restorations were etched with hydrochloric acid (Tri-Dynamics Gel for Ceramics, Patterson Dental, St Paul, MN, USA) before being delivered for insertion.

PHASE 3: INSERTION

Upon delivery from the laboratory (Americus Dental Laboratory, DSG) the restorations were examined on the master cast for fit, integrity, accuracy, and consistency of shade (**Fig. 12**).

The patient was given appointment to return; the provisionals were removed; preparations were cleaned, rinsed, and dried; and the restorations were tried in. OptraGate (Ivoclar, Amherst, NY) was placed in order to retract the lips and keep a controlled, moisture-free, uncontaminated field. The restorations were tried in with water placed on the internal aspect of the veneers. This step allowed the visualization of the margin integrity, fit, contour, length, and shade of all restorations before inserting them permanently. The parameters were evaluated, and it was determined that the shade did not require any alteration for insertion, so translucent shade of luting resin (Choice 2, BISCO, Inc, Schaumburg, IL, USA) was used to place the restorations.

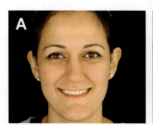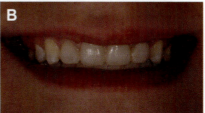

Fig. 11. (*A*) Provisionals full face. (*B*) Provisionals smile.

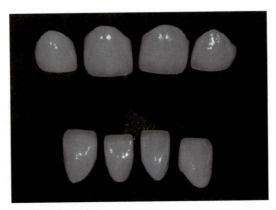

Fig. 12. Restorations before insertion.

The restorations were cleaned with phosphoric acid 35% (Ultradent Products, Inc, South Jordan, UT, USA) for 20 seconds. Each restoration was previously etched by the laboratory; this was to remove any debris on the restorations that may have occurred during try in. The restorations were silinated (BIS-SILANE Part 1 & 2, BISCO, Inc), and a thin coat of porcelain bonding resin (Choice 2) was placed in on the intaglio surface of the veneers, and covered, while the teeth were prepared for the bonding process. The teeth were etched with 35% phosphoric acid (Ultradent Products, Inc) for 20 seconds. ALL-BOND Part I and 2 (BISCO, Inc) were combined, applied to the teeth, and air-thinned. Choice 2 Translucent Luting Resin (Bisco, Schaumburg, IL) was applied to the restorations and the restorations were placed on the teeth. The excess was cleaned with bristle brushes, and the restorations were light-tacked at the gingival margins (VALO Curing Light, Ultradent Products, Inc). The excess was flossed away, and the restorations were light-cured for 45 seconds. The occlusion was adjusted accordingly. The restorations were polished, and the incisal edges were recontoured slightly. The patient returned postoperatively to make any further adjustments and for photographs to be taken (**Fig. 13**).

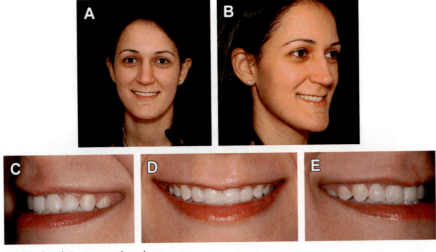

Fig. 13. (*A–E*) Postoperative views.

PHASE 4: MAINTENANCE

It is important for the restorative dentist to think about postorthodontic retention. It was decided that the best form of retention would be an Essix retainer (Dentsply) fabricated after the completion of the restorative treatment. On the mandibular arch, a lingual arch wire was bonded from canine to canine.

DISCUSSION

Minimally invasive esthetic dentistry requires a thorough understanding of smile design and function. By using the NYUCD Smile Evaluation Form, it was possible to formulate an interdisciplinary treatment plan to achieve a minimally invasive esthetic result that is also functional. An interdisciplinary modality of treatment involves communication between the restorative dentist and specialists involved with the case. It is imperative for there to be a dialogue regarding the course of treatment. The restoring dentist has the responsibility to coordinate all treatment to achieve the best clinical outcome. As in the case presented, a midtreatment modification to the treatment plan was necessary to achieve the desired result. All clinicians, as well as the patient, were involved in the decision-making process. By following the principles of smile design it was possible to achieve an esthetic result with the least amount of tooth structure being removed.

RESULTS AND SUMMARY

Postoperatively, the maxillary dental midlines coincide with the facial midline. The axial inclinations of the treated teeth are close to ideal. The patient has a full buccal corridor. All spaces have been closed. The patient has a Class I canine relationship on both the right and left sides. Adequate overbite and overjet have been achieved. There is an overall facial esthetic improvement with the restorations that have been placed. The restorations are both functional and esthetic and fulfill the patient's initial chief concern.

ACKNOWLEDGMENTS

The Authors would like to acknowledge DSG Americus Dental Labrotory and Oleg Gorlenko MDT for the hard work and dedication to achieving aesthetic excellence in this case.

REFERENCES

1. Calamia JR, Levine JB, Lipp M, et al. Smile design and treatment planning with the help of a comprehensive esthetic evaluation form. Dent Clin North Am 2011;55(2): 187–210.
2. Evaluating facial esthetics: the esthetic plane. Frank Spear Daily Digest. Available at: http://www.speareducation.com/. Accessed August, 2014.
3. Kokich VO Jr, Kiyak HA, Shapiro PA. Comparing the perception of dentists and lay people to altered dental esthetics. J Esthet Dent 1999;11(6):311–24.
4. Chu SJ, Tan JH, Stappert CF, et al. Gingival zenith positions and levels of the maxillary anterior dentition. J Esthet Restor Dent 2009;21(2):113–20.
5. Gurel G. Porcelain laminate veneers: minimal tooth preparation by design. Dent Clin North Am 2007;51:419–31, ix.
6. Calamia JR, Calamia CS. Porcelain laminate veneers: reasons for 25 years of success. Dent Clin North Am 2007;51:399–417, ix.
7. LeSage B, Wells D. Myths vs realities: two viewpoints on prepared veneers and prep-less veneers. J Cosmet Dentistry 2011;27(2):66–76.

The Interplay of Orthodontics, Periodontics, and Restorative Dentistry to Achieve Aesthetic and Functional Success

Richard D. Trushkowsky, DDS[a],*, Zainab Alsadah, BDS[b],
Luis M. Brea, DDS[a], Anabella Oquendo, DDS[a]

KEYWORDS

• Orthodontics • Periodontics • Restorative dentistry • Esthetics • Functionality

KEY POINTS

- Previously dentists focused on repair and maintenance of function.
- The emphasis of many patients and dentists is now on esthetics.
- Often there is a need for the disciplines of orthodontics, periodontics, restorative dentistry, and maxillofacial surgery to work together in order to achieve optimum results.
- Currently the planning process begins with esthetics and then function, structure, and ultimately biology.

The past 20 to 30 years have seen substantial changes in the practice of dentistry. In admittedly economically advantaged populations, the daily routine has largely shifted from the unrelenting need to repair the ravages of disease to one of providing elective and to large extent cosmetic services. One could, perhaps, ascribe this change to the advent of sealants, fluorides, and the awareness of the role of bacteria in causing decay and periodontal disease.[1] Whatever the cause, the condition of the mouth can have a strong impact on a patient's psychological, social, and functional health.[2]

The authors have nothing to disclose.
[a] Advanced Program for International Dentists in Aesthetic Dentistry, Department of Cariology and Comprehensive Care, New York University College of Dentistry, 345 East 24th Street, Clinic 7W, New York, NY 10010, USA; [b] Advanced Program for International Dentists in Aesthetic Dentistry, New York University College of Dentistry, 345 East 24th Street, Clinic 7W, New York, NY 10010, USA
* Corresponding author.
E-mail address: Rt587@nyu.edu

dental.theclinics.com

To optimize outcomes, there is often a need to integrate the disciplines of orthodontics, periodontics, restorative dentistry, and maxillofacial surgery. Improvement in esthetic satisfaction due to orthodontic or orthodontic-surgical treatment seems to lead to improvement in oral health and related quality of life. Sarver and Ackerman recommended ascertaining the positive characteristics of a patient's smile to be sure that one shields the patient as treatment is directed at the more challenging aspects. A visualized treatment strategy must then be created to address the patient's chief concerns.[3] But in the end it is the restorative practitioner who is responsible for the final case outcome. Therefore an appreciation of the dental disciplines required to plan a properly sequenced treatment plan is essential. An increasing number of adult orthodontic patients who present with periodontal problems have been reported.[4] The orthodontic problems that can often be found in patients with periodontal involvement include: proclination of the maxillary anterior teeth, irregular dental spacing, rotation, overeruption, migration, loss of teeth, or traumatic occlusion. Orthodontics in conjunction with periodontal treatment can often add considerably to the esthetic outcome. It is both intellectually interesting and a challenge to traditional values that efficacious contemporary sequential treatment planning philosophy begins with esthetics. Function, structure, and ultimately biology must then be incorporated into the planning. To treat a patient solely on the basis of esthetic outcome is an open invitation to long-term failure.

CASE REPORT

The patient is a 53-year-old female professional singer. Her chief complaint revolved around old composite restorations that "make my front teeth appear darker" and made her unhappy with her smile. She expressed a desire to straighten her bottom teeth, whiten her upper teeth, have a better curvature of her upper teeth and for her mouth to appear more attractive. A medical history was taken, and a caries risk assessment and a comprehensive extraoral examination and intraoral examination were conducted.

Dental History

Occlusal composite restorations had been done on teeth #2, #3, #4, #5, #15, #18, #19, #30, and #31; distal-occlusal (DO) composite on tooth #5; and mesial composites only on teeth #8 and #9. Gingival recession was approximately 3 mm on teeth #10 and #11. The New York University College of Dentistry (NYUCD) smile evaluation form was utilized to evaluate the patient's chief complaint and to provide macroesthetic and microesthetic information required to make a correct diagnosis and formulate a treatment plan that would address the patient's concerns.

Upon completion of the smile analysis, the following problems were noted:

The patient's dental maxillary midline was deviated and canted to the left.
Her lower midline was deviated to the right.
There were crowded lower anteriors.
There was proclination of the maxillary anteriors.
3 mm gingival recession on #'s 10 and 11 were noted.
A minimal amount of tooth structure was displayed at rest (**Fig. 1**).
A reverse smile was present (**Fig. 2**).

Orthodontic, periodontal, and restorative therapies were indicated in order to address all of the patient's needs.

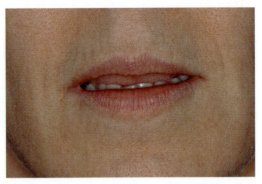

Fig. 1. Rest position demonstrated no visibility of maxillary incisors.

Diagnostic Aids

A full series of radiographs revealed recurrent caries under old composites on teeth #8, #9, and #11. Subsequently a full series of photographs was obtained in accordance with the guidelines established for the Advanced Program for International Dentists in Aesthetic Dentistry. Impressions were obtained with Reprosil (Dentsply Caulk, Milford, Delaware) for study models. A face bow record (Artex, Amann Girrbach AG, Koblach, Austria) and centric bite (Blu-*Bite* HP, Henry Schein, Melville, New York) were obtained to mount the study casts on a semiadjustable articulator (Artex) (**Fig. 3**). A wax-up was fabricated based upon biomimetic principles and influenced by patient input. A putty index (Coltene Lab-Putty, Coltène/Whaledent Incorporated, Cuyahoga Falls, Ohio) was fabricated from the wax-up and an intraoral mock-up was done with a Bis-acryl material (Luxatemp Ultra, DMG America, Englewood, New Jersey) (**Fig. 4**) so that the patent could visualize the final esthetic design. After discussion with the patient and laboratory, it was decided that feldspathic porcelain veneers from teeth #5 through #12 would achieve the patient's desires. Because the patient desired lighter teeth, bleaching of the mandibular anterior teeth was to be completed after the veneer placement (Zoom, Philips Oral Healthcare, Stamford, Connecticut). Restorations fabricated using E Max (Ivoclar, Vivadent, Amherst, New York) were considered. After consultation with the laboratory technician, the authors jointly decided that feldspathic porcelain was the material of choice, as the preparations could be less invasive and result in veneers with superior optical qualities.

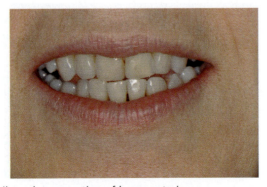

Fig. 2. Reverse smile and overeruption of lower anteriors.

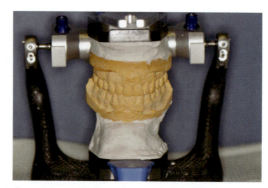

Fig. 3. Cast mounted on Artex articulator in centric relation.

TREATMENT SEQUENCE
Orthodontic Considerations

The patient underwent Invisalign (Align Technology, San Jose, CA) treatment in the NYUCD Orthodontic Department. The goals were to correct the midline, procline the incisors, reduce the open bite in the right molar area, and intrude teeth #8 and #9. Invisalign uses a series of aligners created for the patient that are based upon proprietary computer program projections of the movement of the teeth over 2-week intervals. These aligner trays are worn over the teeth and gradually move them into predicted places. The authors believed that the positions of the teeth following orthodontics would permit more conservative preparation while providing the space required for veneer fabrication. The maxillary central incisors' vertical position is critical in determining the smile arc.[5] Ideally, the upper anterior incisal edges should be coincident with or follow the contour of the lower lip when smiling. After proper alignment of the maxillary anteriors (the new incisal edge position), the length-to-width ratio of the teeth can be considered to maximize the esthetics. The patient was an Angle Class I with 2 mm overjet and 1 to 2 mm overbite. No crowding was present in the maxillary arch, but there was a 3 mm space deficiency in the mandibular arch. Interproximal reduction (IPR) was utilized in the lower arch to create the required space.

Periodontal Considerations

Subsequent to scaling and root planning, the patient had a subepithelial connective tissue graft taken from the palate (**Fig. 5**), with a full-thickness coronally positioned

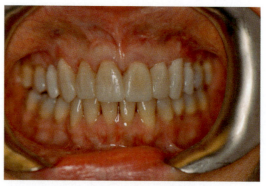

Fig. 4. Intraoral mock-up was done with a Bis-acryl material.

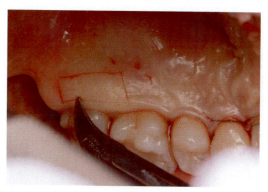

Fig. 5. Subepithelial connective tissue graft taken from the palate.

flap to correct the recession around teeth #10 and #11 (**Fig. 6**). Preoperative intraoral antisepsis was achieved using 0,12% chlorhexidine digluconate solution (Colgate, New York, New York; Perioguard) rinsed for 1 minute. Prior to surgery, the root was lightly scaled with Gracey curettes (Hu-Friedy Manufacturing Company, Chicago, Illinois). The root surfaces were then conditioned with EDTA gel pH 6.70 (Straumann Pregel, Straumann, Basel, Switzerland) for 2 minutes to remove the smear layer, and the visible root was rinsed with copious amounts of sterile saline to remove all the EDTA remaining. This allowed the gingival margins to be symmetric prior to the restorative phase. Two oblique, divergent beveled incisions were made at the bordering teeth and were directed apically in the alveolar mucosa. A split-full thickness flap was used. A passive flap coronal mobilization needs to be achieved at the level of the cemento-enamel junction. The subepithelial connective tissue graft (SCTG) was obtained from the palatal area (see **Fig. 5**). The enamel matrix derivative (EMD) gel was then placed over the root surface, and the SCTG was placed over the gel at the level of the cemento-enamel junction. The graft was trimmed as needed to allow its extension over the bone apically and laterally 2.0 to 3.0 mm (**Fig. 7**). The flap was then positioned coronally 2 mm past the cemento-enamel junction so as to completely cover the graft after suturing **Fig. 8**. The graft enabled a more ideal crown length and gingival height compared with the contralateral side (**Fig. 9**).

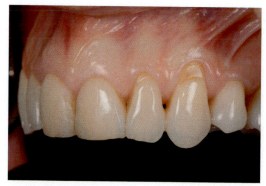

Fig. 6. Recession labial #10 and #11.

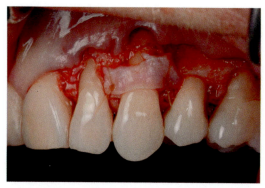

Fig. 7. The graft was trimmed as needed to allow its extension over the bone apically and laterally 2.0–3.0 mm.

Restorative Considerations

To provide the correct macrotooth and microtooth proportions, the treatment plan called for porcelain veneers on teeth 5–12. The proposed tooth sizes and proportions were derived from the wax-up and had been confirmed with an intraoral mock-up. Incisal and labial reduction guides were fabricated using Coltene Lab-Putty (**Figs. 10** and **11**) (Coltène/Whaledent Incorporated, Cuyahoga Falls, Ohio). High-strength feldspathic porcelain was used for the fabrication of the definitive restorations (**Figs. 12–14**). The veneers were cemented with resin cement using only the light-cured base paste. (Variolink II Ivoclar Vivadent, Amherst New York) (**Figs. 15** and **16**). Omitting the chemical cure component permitted more working time and allowed for easier cleanup. The final esthetic results achieved (**Figs. 17–20**) demonstrated the result obtainable with coordination of different dental disciplines. Bleaching of the mandibular dentition allowed matching of the restored maxillary teeth (**Fig. 21**).

DISCUSSION

The desire of patients to improve their appearance has created a need for the restorative clinician to develop a logical diagnostic and treatment approach. However, only

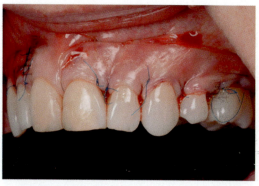

Fig. 8. Full-thickness coronally positioned flap to correct the recession around 10 and 11.

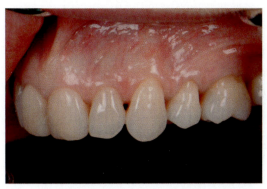

Fig. 9. The graft enabled a more ideal crown length and gingival height compared with the contralateral.

one of the goals in esthetic dentistry should be an improved and natural appearance. An appropriate treatment must also provide the patient with healthy tissues, comfort, efficient mastication, phonetics, and the prospect of long-term survival. To achieve these multiple goals, a team approach that includes multiple dental disciplines may be required. The restorative dentist must have a comprehensive understanding of the benefits each discipline so as to create the corrections required to restore esthetics, biology, and function.

Esthetic evaluation and treatment planning always begin with determining the appropriateness of the incisal edge position of the maxillary centrals relative to the upper lip at rest. If the incisal edge display is inadequate, it will have to be increased. Restorative dentistry, orthodontic extrusion, or a combination of both may be appropriate. If the incisal edge display is excessive, the maxillary incisors need to be moved apically through equilibration, restoration, or orthodontics.[6] The lip line is the quantity of tooth display during smiling. Ideally the lip line (upper lip) should approximate the gingival margin and expose the entire cervicoincisal length of the maxillary central incisors. A high lip line exposes the entire clinical crown and adjacent gingival tissue. A low lip line patient will display less than 75% of the maxillary anterior teeth. The next element that needs to be evaluated is the maxillary dental midline. It has been demonstrated that deviations of 3 to 4 mm are not discerned by lay people when the long axis of the teeth is parallel to the long axis of the

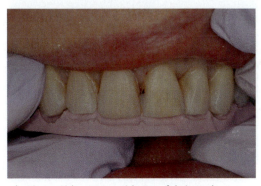

Fig. 10. An incisal reduction guide putty guide was fabricated.

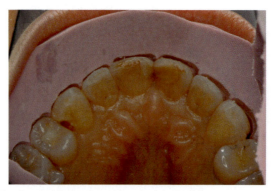

Fig. 11. Labial reduction guide putty guide was fabricated.

face.[7] However, incisors that are canted to the right or left by 2 mm are generally considered unaesthetic. The canting can be corrected by orthodontics, restorative dentistry or a combination of both as was accomplished for this patient. Orthodontics prior to restoration can often minimize tooth reduction. The labiolingual inclination of the maxillary central incisors in relation to the maxillary posterior occlusal plane must be assessed. Ideally, the labial surface of the maxillary central incisors should be perpendicular to the posterior occlusal plane. Correction of the labiolingual inclination may require orthodontics (as was done in this case), restorative correction, or sometimes endodontics.[8]

Determination of the maxillary occlusal plane in comparison to the ideal incisal edge position should be considered. Correction of the posterior occlusal plane may involve orthognathic surgery, restorative procedures, or a combination of both.[6] The determination of gingival levels depends on the preferred tooth size in relation to the incisal edge position. Ideally, the length-to-width ratio of the maxillary anterior teeth is then determined followed by the amount of gingival display desired. If the gingival levels create a short tooth relative to the incisal edge position, the gingival margins need to be moved apically. Selection of the correct procedures depends on the sulcus depth, position of the cemento-enamel junction in relation to the bone level, and the remaining tooth structure compared with the root length and shape.

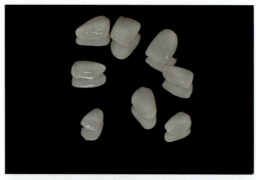

Fig. 12. High-strength feldspathic porcelain was used for the fabrication of the definitive restorations.

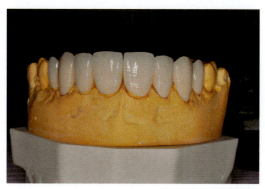

Fig. 13. Veneers on die model demonstrate contour and texture of labial surface.

The lips frame the teeth and gingiva. With the gingiva framing the teeth, the gingival line for anterior teeth should be parallel to the horizon and symmetric.[9] In the case presented here, the gingiva framed the teeth, and the patient had recession in the #10 and #11 area that required surgical coverage to create a symmetric gingival architecture. The elements often associated with recessions are inflammatory periodontal disease, traumatic tooth brushing, and inadequate attached gingival dimensions.[10] This patient had a subepithelial connective tissue graft in conjunction with an EMD placed in the #10 and #11 position. The primary goal of root coverage procedures is to restore tissue esthetics and stability. If support can be regained, that is an added benefit. EMD, used in this case, contains a bone sialoprotein-like molecule that attaches to the human periodontal ligament cell and causes endogenous production of growth factors that promotes periodontal regeneration.[10]

A variety of surgical procedures have been used to achieve root coverage. Subepithelial connective tissue grafting (SCTG) offers a high degree of probability when used to treat Miller's class I and II gingival recession.[10] However, good outcomes have also been obtained using enamel matrix derivative (EMD) in conjunction with coronally advanced flaps and the results appears stable, clinically effective, and similar to each other on all measured parameters.[11] Alkan and Partar also demonstrated that both coronally advanced flap (CAF) + EMD and CAF + CTG procedures were similarly successful in treating Miller Class I and Class II single gingival recession defects.[12] EMD is an amelogenin derivative acquired from porcine embryogenesis and is able to encourage regenerative developments in periodontal tissues as it contains a bone sialoprotein-like moleculec that adheres to the human periodontal ligament cell.

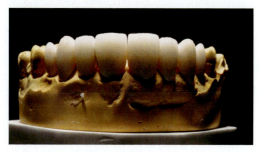

Fig. 14. Light transmission through the porcelain veneers.

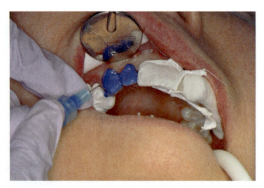

Fig. 15. Isolation with plumbers' tape prior to etching.

This allows the formation of endogenous growth factors conducive to periodontal regeneration.[10]

The papilla levels should then be evaluated. It has been determined by Chu and colleagues[13] that papilla proportions (papilla height to crown length) were approximately 40% for all tooth groups (maxillary anterior teeth). However, Pattil and Desai found papilla proportions were approximately 44% for all tooth groups.[14] Contacts shorter than the papilla would indicate modest-to-substantial incisor abrasion, resulting in shorter crowns and shorter contacts. Altered passive or altered active eruption of teeth can result in significantly longer contacts compared with papilla length. Correction may be required necessitating orthodontic intrusion, extrusion, or osseous surgery in order to refine papilla levels. Discussing tooth shape and shade with the patient is appropriate prior to a diagnostic wax-up. Composite resin can be used intraorally to help ascertain the patient's preferences. An impression of the desired changes could then be taken and the gleaned information incorporated into the wax-up. Once the wax-up is completed, a silicone index can be created.

Porcelain veneers have demonstrated long-term viability, and acceptance by patients.[15] Highton and colleagues[16] stated that incisal reduction allows adequate stress distribution and may provide improved longevity for the veneers. However, others designs have been recommended, and Wall and colleagues[17] and Meijering and colleagues[18] did not find any variance in failure rates between incisal preparation designs. However, an overlapping veneer preparation is required when esthetics of the incisal edge or occlusion require it. Castelnuovo and colleagues[19] found in their

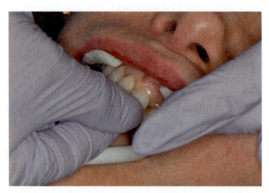

Fig. 16. Placement of each veneer with a light-cured composite resin.

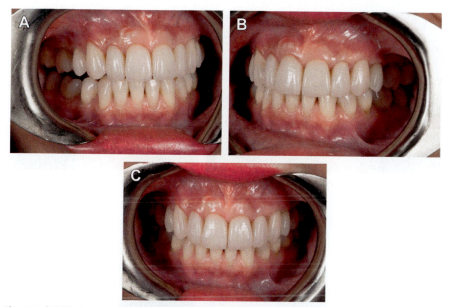

Fig. 17. (*A*) Right lateral view bonded veneers. (*B*) Left lateral view bonded veneers. (*C*) Retracted view demonstrates excellent esthetics and morphology of the veneers.

study that no incisal reduction, or a 2 mm incisal reduction, without palatal chamfer (butt joint) recorded the greatest fracture loads that were comparable to an unrestored control. The butt joint was the type of preparation used for the patient in this case study and is the one usually utilized in the authors' esthetic program for most clinical cases. In addition, the ideal preparation depth and the amount of enamel required have different proponents. In actuality, requirements for each case may vary. Tooth color, shade desired, position in the arch, rotation, and existing restoration such as those in the present case study require modification of the ideal preparation. The preparation should be all in enamel, as it provides the best bond, and its rigidity reduces the risk of ceramic fracture. Although the silicone templates should be used to verify adequate tooth reduction, slight shifting of the guides from precise placement can lead to inadequate or too much preparation.[20]

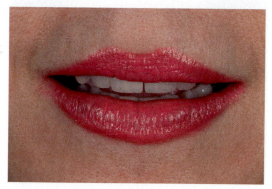

Fig. 18. Incisal edge in repose demonstrates ideal exposure of maxillary anterior teeth.

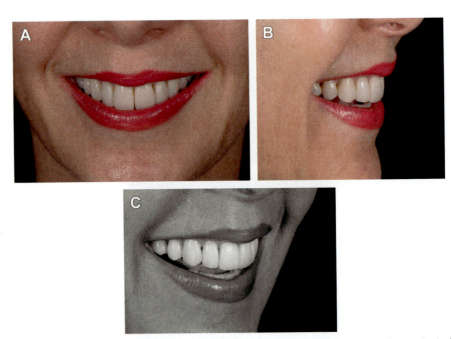

Fig. 19. (*A*) Incisal edge in relation to wet-dry line during smiling. (*B*) Lateral view incisal edge in relation to wet-dry line during smiling. (*C*) Incisal edge in relation to wet-dry line during smiling and posterior occlusal plane.

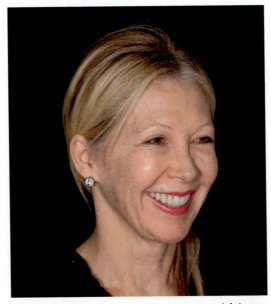

Fig. 20. Esthetic results provides the patient with a more youthful appearance.

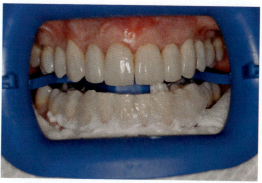

Fig. 21. Bleaching of lower anteriors to correlate with maxillary veneers.

SUMMARY

In order to maximize outcomes that not only enhance esthetics, are stable over the long term, and contribute to the patient's oral health, it is sometimes necessary to adopt a properly sequenced interdisciplinary approach as was done with the patient described in this article.

ACKNOWLEDGMENT

The authors wish to thank Peter Pizzi CDT, MDT- Pizzi Dental Studio, Staten Island, New York, for his contributions in the planning of this case and for fabricating the porcelain veneers.

REFERENCES

1. Spear FM, Kokich VG, Mathews DP. Interdisciplinary management of anterior dental esthetics. J Am Dent Assoc 2006;137:160–9.
2. Silvola AS, Varimo M, Tolvanen M, et al. Dental esthetics and quality of life in adults with severe malocclusion before and after treatment. Angle Orthod 2014;84:594–9.
3. Sarver DM, Ackerman MB. Dynamic smile visualization and quantification: part 1. Evolution of the concept and dynamic records for smile capture. Am J Orthod Dentofacial Orthop 2003;124:4–12.
4. Gkantidis N, Christou P, Topouzelis N. The orthodontic–periodontic interrelationship in integrated treatment challenges: a systematic review. J Oral Rehabil 2010;37:377–90.
5. Sarver DM, Ackerman MB. Dynamic smile visualization and quantification: part 2. Smile analysis and treatment strategies. Am J Orthod Dentofacial Orthop 2003; 124:116–27.
6. Spear FM, Kokich VG. A multidisciplinary approach to esthetic dentistry. Dent Clin North Am 2007;51(2):487–505.
7. Kokich V. Esthetics and anterior tooth position: an orthodontic perspective. Part III: Mediolateral relationships. J Esthet Dent 1993;5:200–7.
8. Spear FM. The esthetic correction of anterior dental mal-alignment conventional vs. instant (restorative) orthodontics. J Calif Dent Assoc 2004;32:133–41.
9. McClaren EA, Cao PT. Smile analysis and esthetic design: "in the zone." Inside Dentistry 2009;5:44–8.

10. Henriques PS, Pelegrine AA, Nogueira AA, et al. Application of subepithelial connective tissue graft with or without enamel matrix derivative for root coverage: a split-mouth randomized study. J Oral Sci 2010;52:463–71.

11. McGuire MK, Scheyer ET, Nunn M. Evaluation of human recession defects treated with coronally advanced flaps and either enamel matrix derivative or connective tissue: comparison of clinical parameters at 10 years. J Periodontol 2012; 83:1353–62.

12. Alkan EA, Parlar A. EMD or subepithelial connective tissue graft for the treatment of single gingival recessions: a pilot study. J Periodontal Res 2011;46:637–42.

13. Chu SJ, Tarnow DP, Tan JH, et al. Papilla proportions in the maxillary anterior dentition. Int J Periodontics Restorative Dent 2009;29:385–93.

14. Patil VA, Desai MH. Assessment of gingival contours for esthetic diagnosis and treatment: a clinical study. Indian J Dent Res 2013;24:394–5.

15. Stappert CF, Stathopoulou N, Gerds T, et al. Survival rate and fracture strength of maxillary incisors, restored with different kinds of full veneers. J Oral Rehabil 2005;32:266–72.

16. Highton R, Caputo AA, Mátyás J. A photoelastic study of stresses on porcelain laminate preparations. J Prosthet Dent 1987;58:157–61.

17. Wall JG, Reisbick MH, Espeleta KG. Cement luting thickness beneath porcelain veneers made on platinum foil. J Prosthet Dent 1992;68:448–50.

18. Meijering AC, Roeters FJ, Mulder J, et al. Patients' satisfaction with different types of veneer restorations. J Dent 1997;25:493–7.

19. Castelnuovo J, Tjan AH, Phillips K, et al. Fracture load and mode of failure of ceramic veneers with different preparations. J Prosthet Dent 2000;83:171–80.

20. Hajtó J, Marinescu C. An esthetic challenge: isolated areas of high translucency in laminate veneers. Eur J Esthet Dent 2012;7:282–94.

Treatment of the Patient with Gummy Smile in Conjunction with Digital Smile Approach

David Montalvo Arias, DDS[a], Richard D. Trushkowsky, DDS[a],*,
Luis M. Brea, DDS[b], Steven B. David, DMD[b]

KEYWORDS

• Gummy smile • Gingival display • Crown length • Porcelain veneers

KEY POINTS

• Gummy smile cases are always esthetically demanding cases.

• This article presents a case treated with an interdisciplinary treatment approach and Digital Smile Approach (DSA) using Keynote (DSA), to predictably achieve an esthetic outcome for a patient with gummy smile.

• In order to formulate a treatment plan that predictably leads to a successful esthetic outcome, the final appearance of the case must be visualized and defined before the initiation of active treatment.

• The importance of using questionnaires and checklists to facilitate the gathering of diagnostic data cannot be overemphasized.

• The acquired data must then be transferred to the design of the final restorations.

• The use of digital smile design has emerged as a powerful tool in cosmetic dentistry to help both the practitioner and the patient visualize the final outcome.

INTRODUCTION

A smile's attractiveness is determined by tooth shapes, position, and color, as well as the extent and healthy appearance of the gingival tissue display. The overall relationship between these elements and the face complete the esthetic determinants.

The authors have nothing to disclose.
[a] Advanced Program for International Dentists in Aesthetic Dentistry, NYU College of Dentistry, New York, NY, USA; [b] Advanced Program for International Dentists in Aesthetic Dentistry, Department of Cariology and Comprehensive Care, NYU College of Dentistry, New York, NY, USA
* Corresponding author.
E-mail address: Rt587@nyu.edu

Dent Clin N Am 59 (2015) 703–716
http://dx.doi.org/10.1016/j.cden.2015.03.007
0011-8532/15/$ – see front matter © 2015 Elsevier Inc. All rights reserved.

dental.theclinics.com

Computer design software has evolved into the major component of the communication between dentists, technicians, and patients. The power of digital technology can now be incorporated into the smile design procedure. Although there are several proprietary digital design services available in the marketplace (Smile Designer Pro, Toronto, Ontario, Canada; Digital Smile Design, Sao Paulo, Brazil). Photoshop software (Adobe Systems, San Jose, CA, USA), PowerPoint (Microsoft Corp, Redmond, WA, USA), or Keynote (Apple Inc, Cupertino, CA, USA) can also be used to facilitate patient input, conceptualization of outcomes, and laboratory communication. The design must be based upon an understanding of macroesthetic and microesthetic concepts regardless of the system used.[1,2] The primary author used Keynote (as others have done) with a DSA to create a smile design incorporating correction of the patient's chief complaint and information derived from the New York University (NYU) esthetic evaluation form.

Soft tissue surgical periodontal plastic procedures play an important role in the enhancement of smile by helping to optimize the relationships between the 3 primary components: the teeth, the lip framework, and the gingival scaffold.[3] Kois[4] has stated that when attempting to enhance esthetic outcomes, the influence of 2 essential biological concerns must be fully understood. The first, location of the base of the sulcus, influences the cervical termination of tooth preparation and allows for intracrevicular location of the restoration margin. The second, knowledge of location of the osseous crest, is required before altering gingival levels. The so-called gummy smile is largely a result of an unfavorable ratio between upper lip length and gingiva/tooth display. The location of the smile line is also essentially the product of this ratio. The smile line is defined as the ratio between the upper lip and visibility of the gingival tissue and teeth. Smile level is an imaginary line that follows the lower margin of the upper lip and usually has a convex appearance.[5] Cases exhibiting excessively short teeth and a lack of tooth display are frequently encountered esthetic problems. Excessive gingival display may also be encountered in cases with short teeth. When the incisal edge position is correct, crown lengthening can be used to increase the clinical crown length as a stand-alone esthetic procedure. When the incisal edge position is inadequate and there is excessive gingival display, crown lengthening in conjunction with restorative treatment is indicated. The surgical technique involves apically positioning the gingival margin and may require the removal of supporting bone. The periodontal surgical procedure must also result in a proper biological width and adequate keratinized tissue. Gummy smile can also be the result of altered passive eruption (the alveolar crest is <2 mm from the cementoenamel junction), gingival overgrowth,[6] inadequate length of the upper lip, muscular hyperelevation of the upper lip, and vertical maxillary excess.[7,8] Cases in which there has been extrusion of the upper teeth, with an associated deep bite, present a related problem.[9]

The initial step in establishing a correct diagnosis and a definitive plan of treatment is through a proper classification of the gingival level. Tjan and colleagues[10] established the smile guidelines standards in the 1980s. Smiles were classified into 3 basic categories (high, average, and low) depending on the exposure of the midfacial cervical margin of the clinical crown relative to the vermillion border. This article shows a step-by-step procedure describing how to optimize the final esthetic outcome with the aid of the digital smile design approach and the proper steps to follow in the diagnosis and treatment planning of a patient with gummy smile.

CASE PRESENTATION

The patient, a Latin American homemaker in her mid-50s, presented with the chief complaint of wanting to improve her appearance. Specifically she sought dental treatment because she did not like her front teeth and desired to improve her smile (**Figs. 1–3**).

A medical history was taken, and a comprehensive extraoral and intraoral examination was conducted. The patient had an extensive previous dental history, including crowns, composite restorations, and root canals. An esthetic evaluation of the patient was also performed. This evaluation included mounted models, radiographs, photographs, and an esthetic evaluation form incorporating the changes desired by the patient.

The following problem list was created from the gathered data:

- Localized initial periodontitis (No. 2–3 and No. 6–7)
- Caries No. 2, 3, 5, 13, 19, and 31
- Poorly filled root canals No. 2, 7, and 8
- Overeruption No. 8 and 9
- Excessive maxillary gingival display
- Abrasion No. 21 to 28
- Poor-fitting crowns No. 7, 8, and 9
- A narrow arch form.

Determination of the origin of the problem is extremely important in patients presenting with a gummy smile, which can be skeletal, muscular, dentogingival, or a combination of several or more factors. Knowing the origin of the problem helps to guide the treatment decisions.

Initially, a healthy oral environment was achieved by oral hygiene instruction; localized scaling and root planning on No. 2–3 and No. 6–7; endodontic re-treatment of No. 2, 7, and 8; and composite restorations on No. 2, 3, 19, and 31.

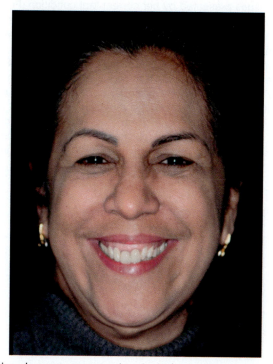

Fig. 1. Full face view demonstrates extensive gingival exposure.

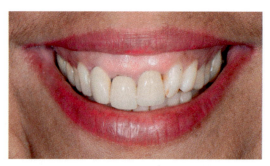

Fig. 2. Smile close-up.

Once hard and soft tissues free of disease were obtained, the final design and position of the restorations were defined by the primary author with the aid of the DSA. The DSA was particularly useful in this case because there was insufficient room for additive mock-up material (usually composite) in the unprepared case. Precisely replicating every detail of the DSA design, strictly adhering to the data flow, enables achievement of the predicted esthetic outcome. A digital caliper was used to measure some reference points on the casts (**Fig. 4**). With the aid of a calibrated virtual digital ruler, the reference points are subsequently transferred to the computer photographs of the patient (**Figs. 5–7**). The newly established incisal edge position, as always, dictated the design of the restorations.

The digitally designed images allowed the patient to visualize the final result and comprehend the issues presented by her current oral condition (**Figs. 8** and **9**). The number of teeth requiring restoration and the need for periodontal surgeries became apparent. The patient's approval to proceed with the treatment was based upon viewing the potential outcome via the DSA software.

The first wax-up was created based on the DSA measurements (**Fig. 10**). The restorations proposed in the wax-up were transferred to the patient's mouth (the mockup) through the use of a silicone putty matrix (Coltene Lab-Putty, Coltène/Whaledent Inc Cuyahoga Falls, OH, USA) and bisacryl (Luxatemp Ultra, DMG America, Englewood, NJ, USA). The incisal edge position and parallelism to the horizontal reference line were verified. A few minor intraoral modifications were made and followed by an impression of the mock-up. Models were poured on which the final wax-up was

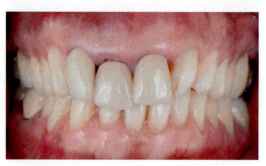

Fig. 3. Retracted intraoral close-up.

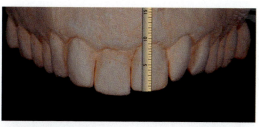

Fig. 4. Calibration of digital ruler on cast.

created. Indexes fabricated from this wax-up were used as the surgical and preparation guides (**Figs. 11–13**).

The esthetic crown lengthening surgery was accomplished, with the aid of the guides, correcting the gingival margin levels. To increase predictability, the procedure was divided into 2 distinct phases. Initially, the old crowns were removed, a mock-up was performed (**Fig. 14**), a gingivectomy was accomplished (**Fig. 15**), and the provisionals were inserted (**Fig. 16**). The biological width was deliberately violated. Dividing the overall periodontal procedure into 2 phases meant shorter appointments and enabled tooth preparation margin position correction. Osseous recontouring to establish an acceptable biological width was accomplished 3 weeks later. A full-thickness flap was raised to allow visualization during the osteoplasty and permit accurate positioning of the gingival margin (**Figs. 17** and **18**).

Six weeks postsurgery, the preparations were modified (**Fig. 19**) and long-term provisionals were placed (Luxatemp). The shape of the provisionals were similar to the contour established in the DSA (**Fig. 20**). Six months postsurgery, final impressions of the prepared teeth were made using retraction cord (Ultrapak, Ultradent Products, Inc, South Jordan, UT, USA) and a polyvinyl siloxane impression material (Aquasil, Dentsply Caulk, Milford, DE, USA). Maximum intercuspation (centric occlusion) bites were recorded (Blu-Bite HP, Henry Schein Inc, Melville, NY, USA). Impressions, bites, clinical pictures, and shades were sent to the laboratory. The models were mounted in centric occlusion on a semiadjustable articulator with a facebow transfer (Artex Articulator System, Amann Girrbach AG, Koblach, Austria).

In consultation with the laboratory, it was decided to fabricate IPS e.max (Ivoclar Vivadent Inc, Amherst, NY, USA) crowns on No. 7, 8, and 9; veneers on No. 6, 10, and 11 in the maxilla; veneers on No. 21 to 27 in the mandible; and onlay veneers

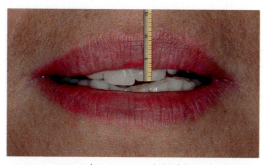

Fig. 5. Calibrated measurement used to measure initial incisal edge exposure.

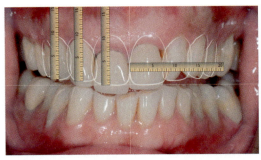

Fig. 6. Calibrated measurements on photograph of maxillary anterior teeth.

on No. 4, 5, 12, and 13. IPS e.max was chosen for both its esthetic qualities and physical properties. After inspection of the ceramics, transparent shade try-in gel was used to position the restorations on the prepared teeth (Variolink II, Ivoclar Vivadent Inc). The patient was given an opportunity to see the restorations in her mouth and gave her consent before their cementation. A water rinse was used to remove all traces of the try-in gel from the restorations. The internal surfaces of the restorations were scrubbed for 15 seconds with a 35% phosphoric acid solution (Ultra-etch, Ultradent Products, Inc) and ultrasonically cleaned in alcohol for 1 minute. Silane primer (Ultradent Products, Inc) was placed on the internal surface of the veneers and allowed to air-dry. Bonding agent (Prime&Bond NT, Dentsply Caulk) was applied and the solvent allowed to evaporate for 30 seconds. The veneered teeth were isolated with rubber dam and Teflon tape, etched with Ultra-etch for 15 seconds, and rinsed with water for 30 seconds. Prime&Bond NT bonding agent was applied to the internal service of the veneers and light-cured for 10 seconds The restorations were then loaded with the base shade of a dual-cured cement (Variolink II cement transparent) and seated on the teeth. A small brush and floss were used to remove the excess cement before light curing for 40 seconds. The crowns were cemented with RelyX Unicem (3M ESPE, St Paul, MN, USA). A final check of the occlusion was made with articulating paper (Accufilm, Parkell Inc, Edgewood, NY, USA), and minor adjustments were performed.

The gummy smile of the patient was not completely corrected, because of its skeletal origin. Other treatment options were offered to the patient, such as orthodontic treatment and orthognathic surgery, but were declined. Despite these

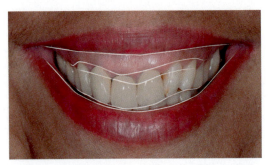

Fig. 7. Lips, gingival margins, papilla height, and incisal edge are delineated.

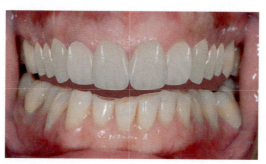

Fig. 8. Intraoral DSA.

limitations, the final result achieved in this case demonstrates what may be accomplished using a systematic interdisciplinary approach assisted by DSA (see **Fig. 20**; **Figs. 21–24**).

DISCUSSION

Esthetically driven restorations for the anterior teeth have become an accepted norm in contemporary dental practice. The esthetic objective affects the treatment planning

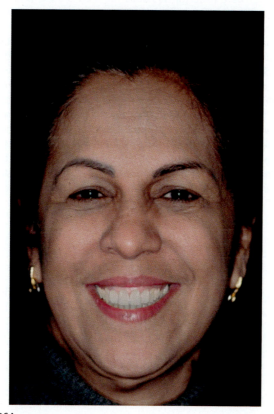

Fig. 9. Full face DSA.

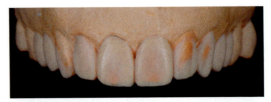

Fig. 10. Initial wax-up based on DSA measurements.

process. The esthetic wax-up is often used to confirm the treatment plan before definitive preparations. Accumulated diagnostic data guide the design of the final restorations. The patient's requirements, within the confines of biological and functional considerations, also need to be incorporated into the final design. Photoshop design software or a variety of commercially available programs can be used before a conventional wax-up to give direction to the process and to communicate with both the patient and the interdisciplinary professional team (the pictures require calibration). Visualization of the final result is accomplished, and the required logical treatment sequence is conceptualized. A series of photographs, as is required in the International Esthetic Program, and an esthetic evaluation form, such as the NYU College of Dentistry esthetic evaluation form, are prerequisites to performing a digital smile design. The DSA software used for this case required 3 basic photographs: full face with a wide smile and teeth apart, full face at rest, and a retracted view with teeth separated. A 45° view and a profile view are also beneficial. A digital facebow is then created by relating the full face smile to horizontal reference lines such as the interpupillary line. A vertical line establishes the midline relying on glabella, nose, and chin as references. On completion, the smile analysis can be concluded. Horizontal lines drawn on the photograph, namely, tip of the canine to contralateral canine, incisal ridge of one central to the incisal edge of contralateral central, and the dental midline, help to calibrate the features presented on the photograph. A digital ruler calibrated against the patient's model is used to measure the width/length percentage of the central incisors. A variety of tooth shapes, available as templates and chosen with patient input, can be inserted.[11] The pink and white evaluation can also be determined as the relationship between the teeth and smile line are readily delineated. All this information is then transferred to a wax-up and subsequently to an intraoral mock-up. This

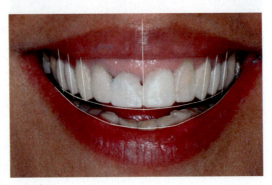

Fig. 11. Incisal edge mock-up.

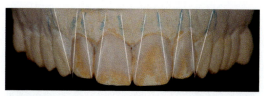

Fig. 12. Final wax-up.

preliminary workup confirmed the need of the patient for esthetic crown lengthening in order to achieve the patient's esthetic goals.

Ideally the amount of gingival display is approximately 1 mm. Excessive gingival display is considered to be more than 3 mm. However, the relationship between gingival and incisor display is a determining factor.[12] As males usually have longer lips, females display more gingiva during maximum smiles.[13,14] Crown lengthening for this patient was esthetically driven and depended on the position of the envisioned incisal edge and the length of the tooth desired.[15,16] Communication between the restorative dentist and the surgeon is required in order to delineate the anticipated tooth position and free gingival margin location. Before surgery, the soft tissue should be measured by sounding to crestal bone in order to approximate the amount of osseous resection required.[17] The surgery can be done in either of the following 2 ways.[18] In the first method, the osseous component is completed with the height of bone placed in the position required to maintain the biological width.[19] The flap is placed back in its original position. After an appropriate healing time, a gingivectomy places the soft tissue in the correct position and reestablishes an acceptable the biological width. The teeth may then be provisionalized. This technique reduces the rebound effect of the soft tissue eliminating the need for more surgery. A second technique requires a gingivectomy, teeth preparation at the new gingival level, and provisionals placed. After that procedure, a full-thickness flap is raised to allow a bone level repositioning by the surgeon with osseous recontouring as needed to re-create adequate biological width. This second technique can be staged into different procedures. In the first stage, gingivectomy and provisionalization are pursued. After a few weeks, the full-thickness flap can be raised to re-create the new apically positioned biological width. Placement of the provisional restorations hinders the formation of the dentogingival complex, but if only allowed to remain for 2 to 4 weeks, it will not provoke an inflammatory reaction. The final gingival margin location and stability depend on the biotype, extent of osteotomy, and flap adaptation. Ideally, a waiting period of 3 months is suggested before proceeding to the final restorative phase. As 2 to 3 mm of keratinized tissue needs to remain after surgery, the amount of keratinized tissue initially present is important. Advantageously, the patient does not have any time during which unappealing roots are exposed.

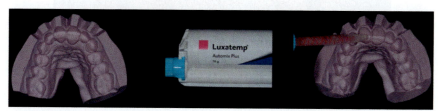

Fig. 13. Mock-up indexes.

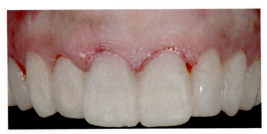

Fig. 14. Mock-up as a surgical stent.

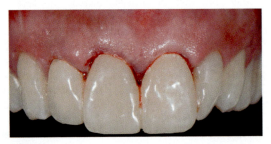

Fig. 15. Gingivectomy and preparation modification.

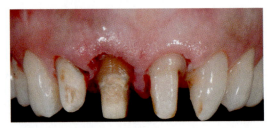

Fig. 16. Provisionalization.

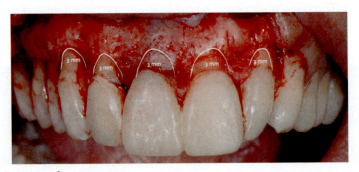

Fig. 17. Exposure of osseous crest.

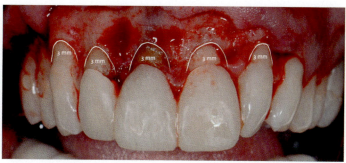

Fig. 18. Bone recontouring.

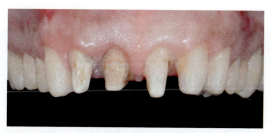

Fig. 19. Final preparations.

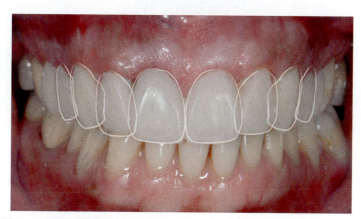

Fig. 20. DSA versus provisionals.

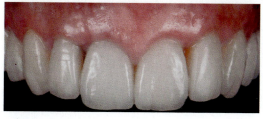

Fig. 21. Final restorations.

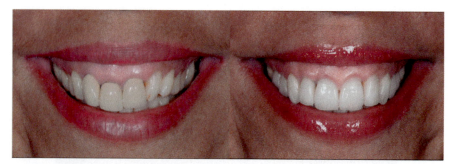

Fig. 22. Smile before and after.

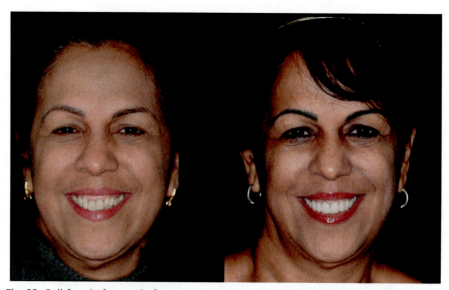

Fig. 23. Full face before and after.

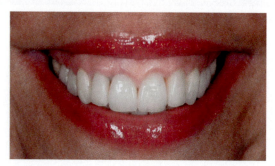

Fig. 24. Final smile close-up.

SUMMARY

The DSA, as used in the case presented here, is a powerful tool for use in esthetic dentistry. DSA is a diagnostic instrument, patient education and marketing tool, education tool for dentists, and an aid in laboratory communication. DSA provides feedback as to the results achievable with minimum restorative dentistry. When exploited to its fullest potential, it provides insights into the predictability of the treatment, reduces mistakes, and allows to control of risk factors (see **Fig. 24**). Optimizing outcomes by assessing the origin of the problems is the key point in determining the need for specialty involvement in the treatment of a patient with gummy smile. Digital visualization of the final outcome and an understanding of the limitations of each treatment procedure guide best practice decisions for a given case.

ACKNOWLEDGMENTS

The authors wish to thank Peter Pizzi, MDT, CDT, of Pizzi Dental Studio for his contributions in the planning of this case and for fabricating the restorations.

REFERENCES

1. McLaren EA, Culp L. Smile analysis - the Photoshop smile design technique: part 1. J Cosmet Dent 2013;29:94–108.
2. McLaren EA, Garber DA, Figueira J. The Photoshop smile design technique (part 1): digital dental photography. Compend Contin Educ Dent 2013;34:772–9.
3. Garber DA, Salama MA. The aesthetic smile: diagnosis and treatment. Periodontol 2000 1996;11:18–28.
4. Kois JC. Altering gingival levels: the restorative connection part I: biologic variables. J Esthet Restor Dent 1994;6:3–7.
5. Oliveira MT, Molina GO, Furtado A, et al. Gummy smile: a contemporary and multidisciplinary overview. Dent Hypotheses 2013;4:55–60.
6. Ong M, Tseng SC, Wang HL. Surgical crown lengthening. Clinic Adv Periodontics 2011;1(3):233–9.
7. Monaco A, Streni O, Marci MC, et al. Gummy smile: clinical parameters useful for diagnosis and therapeutical approach. J Clin Pediatr Dent 2004;29:19–25.
8. Hwang WS, Hur MS, Hu KS, et al. Surface anatomy of the lip elevator muscles for the treatment of gummy smile using botulinum toxin. Angle Orthod 2009;79:70–7.
9. Kim TW, Kim H, Lee SJ. Correction of deep overbite and gummy smile by using a mini-implant with a segmented wire in a growing Class II DIVISION 2 patient. Am J Orthod Dentofacial Orthop 2006;130:676–85.
10. Tjan AH, Miller GD, The JG. Some aesthetic factors in a smile. J Prosthet Dent 1984;51:24–8.
11. Coachman C, Calamita M. Digital Smile Design: A Tool for Treatment Planning and Communication in Esthetic Dentistry. Quintessence Dent Technol 2012;35:103–11.
12. Khan F, Abbas M. Frequency of gingival display during smiling and comparison of biometric measurements in subjects with and without gingival display. J Coll Physicians Surg Pak 2014;24:503–7.
13. Al-Jabrah O, Al-Shammout R, El-Naji W, et al. Gender differences in the amount of gingival display during smiling using two intraoral dental biometric measurements. J Prosthodont 2010;19:286–93.
14. Al-Habahbeh R, Al-Shammout R, Al-Jabrah O, et al. The effect of gender on tooth and gingival display in the anterior region at rest and during smiling. Eur J Esthet Dent 2009;4:382–95.

15. Chu SJ, Hochman MN. A biometric approach to aesthetic crown lengthening: part I–midfacial considerations. Pract Proced Aesthet Dent 2008;20:17–24.
16. Chu SJ, Hochman MN, Fletcher P. A biometric approach to aesthetic crown lengthening: part II–interdental considerations. Pract Proced Aesthet Dent 2008;20:529–36.
17. Perez JR, Smukler H, Nunn ME. Clinical evaluation of the supraosseous gingivae before and after crown lengthening. J Periodontol 2007;78:1023–30.
18. Sonick M. Esthetic crown lengthening for maxillary anterior teeth. Compend Contin Educ Dent 1997;18:807–12.
19. Lee EA. Aesthetic crown lengthening: classification, biologic rationale, and treatment planning considerations. Pract Proced Aesthet Dent 2004;16:769–78.

Interdisciplinary Sequencing of Aesthetic Treatment

Michael Apa, DDS[a,b,*], Brian Chadroff, DDS[c]

KEYWORDS

• Facial analysis • Implant • Facial dehiscence

KEY POINTS

• Communication is important to achieve the ultimate perio-restorative interface.
• Facial aesthetic design was used to aid in the development of an aesthetic blueprint, so that soft and hard tissue discrepancies could be eliminated to improve the restorative aesthetic outcome and minimize patients' facial asymmetry.
• The team approach is essential in achieving ideal aesthetics for an interdisciplinary treatment plan.
• When communication occurs properly, the aesthetic surgery can be considered a surgical component of the restorative therapy.

BACKGROUND

A 40-year-old female patient presented to our office with a chief complaint of pain above the upper right central incisor. Her medical history was noncontributory. On radiographic examination it was determined than an endodontic failure existed including periapical pathology and a buccal fistula (**Fig. 1**). Full mouth charting revealed a stable periodontal status with a localized 8-mm midfacial probing approximating the apex of tooth number 8. Dental examination revealed porcelain laminate veneers on teeth numbers 4 to 13, which had been placed approximately 14 years prior.

AESTHETIC EVALUATION

Traditionally we evaluate patients from the facial perspective, then the smile perspective. Finally, we evaluate individual tooth anatomy for proper aesthetics. Before comprehensive evaluation and esthetic treatment planning, we took digital photographs per the

The authors have nothing to disclose.
[a] Rosenthal Apa Group, New York, NY, USA; [b] Department of Cariology and Comprehensive Care, New York University College of Dentistry, New York, NY, USA; [c] Department of Periodontics and Implant Dentistry, New York University College of Dentistry, New York, NY, USA
* Corresponding author.
E-mail address: doctorapa@yahoo.com

Dent Clin N Am 59 (2015) 717–732
http://dx.doi.org/10.1016/j.cden.2015.04.002   **dental.theclinics.com**
0011-8532/15/$ – see front matter © 2015 Elsevier Inc. All rights reserved.

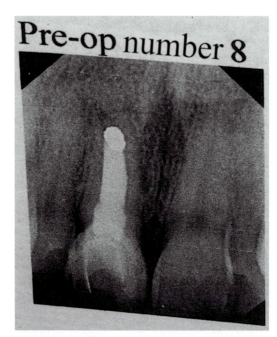

Fig. 1. Initial radiograph of patient.

American Academy of Cosmetic Dentistry's guidelines, and we also took a full mouth series of x-rays, made study models, and performed intraoral charting.

Facial

The patient's facial form is dolichocephalic on visual examination (**Fig. 2**). Both the bridge of the nose and the chin favor the patient's left side. The lower third of the face is the dominant third.

Smile

The patient has existing maxillary veneers from the second premolar to the second premolar (**Fig. 3**). At a full smile the patient shows excessive gingival display with a canting from right to left of the midline (**Fig. 4**). More gingival tissue is shown on the patient's right side than on the left as well as a canting of the existing veneers 4 to 8 to the patient's left. Asymmetrical tissue heights exist both from right of midline to left. Additionally, an asymmetry in tissue height is present between the maxillary centrals. The gingival margin on 8 is approximately 1.5 mm apical to the margin on tooth 9. Convexities appear to be present in the buccal corridor apical to the gingival margins of teeth 3 to 5 and 12 to 14.

Tooth

The narrowness of the patient's facial features dictated that the teeth, especially the central incisors, not be made any longer (**Fig. 5**). However, the angularity of the patient's facial features made it desirable to keep the angular anatomy in the teeth.[1]

PERIODONTAL CONSIDERATIONS

The patient had a chronic endodontic failure of tooth 8, with an existing buccal fistula. From a periodontal perspective, there was minimal overall probing depth except for a

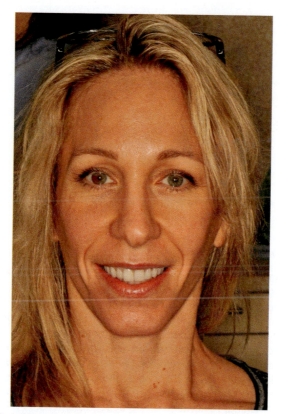

Fig. 2. Patient's facial form is doliochocephalic on visual examination.

localized deep midfacial probing depth on tooth 8 indicating no midfacial bone was present. Although the interproximal bone appeared intact radiographically, there was an existing gingival discrepancy between teeth 8 and 9, with the gingival margin of 8 approximately 1.5 mm apical to 9 (**Fig. 6**). A high smile line existed with associated excessive gingival display from tooth 3 to tooth 8 and tooth 10 to tooth 14. The gingival position of 9 was determined to be ideal in relation to facial aesthetic design and the patient's interpupillary line.

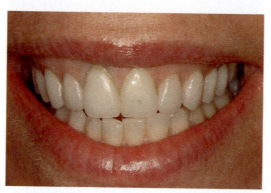

Fig. 3. Patient has existing maxillary veneers from second premolar to second premolar.

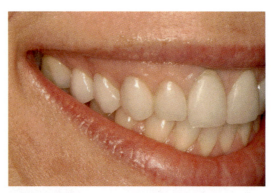

Fig. 4. Right lateral view exhibiting excessive gingival display.

TREATMENT PLAN

The treatment planning for this case required close coordination between restorative and periodontal specialists. Scheduling was critical as the patient would be traveling between two offices during some of the procedures.

The initial treatment plan called for an extraction of the upper right central incisor and an attempt at immediate placement of the implant along with any tissue augmentation that would be required for site development. At the same visit a 2-unit bis-acryl temporary bridge, retained by the left central incisor, would be fabricated. Any additional site development could then be done by removing and adding or subtracting from the provisional. The patient would ultimately require hard and soft tissue crown lengthening, restoration of the upper 10 anteriors (4-7 and 10-13) with porcelain veneers, an implant crown on 8, and a porcelain jacket on 9.

Surgical Treatment

Extraction of 8, implant placement, and temporary bridge

A facial and palatal sulcular incision was performed, and tooth 8 was extracted. A severe facial dehiscence was present approximating the apex of the socket (**Fig. 7**). An

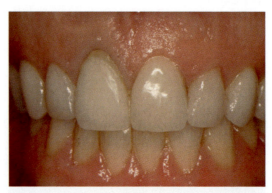

Fig. 5. To compensate for the narrow facial features, the authors elected not to lengthen the central incisors.

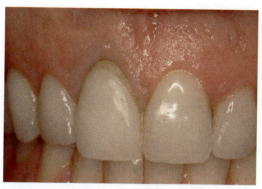

Fig. 6. Patient had an existing gingival discrepancy present between teeth number 8 and number 9, with the gingival margin of number 8 approximately 1.5 mm apical to number 9.

immediate implant[2,3] (Biomet 3i, NanoTite, 5 × 13 mm; Palm Beach Gardens, FL) was stabilized in the residual socket, and demineralized freeze-dried bone allograft (DFDBA; LifeNet Tissue Bank, Virginia Beach, Virginia) was used to fill the gap and augment the facial dehiscence. A thick subepithelial connective tissue graft[4] was used instead of a membrane to augment the soft tissue, improve primary closure, and attempt vertical augmentation that would decrease the existing gingival discrepancy (**Fig. 8**).

The patient then went to the restorative dentist's office for provisionalization. A two-unit cantilever bridge was used with tooth 9 as the abutment. The patient was anesthetized again with 1 carpule of articaine hydrochloride and epinephrine (Septocaine). The existing veneer on tooth 9 was removed carefully so as not to disturb the surgical site. The preparation was continued for a porcelain jacket, with removal of 1.5 mm circumferentially and 1.5 incisally, and scooping out of the lingual surface for prosthetic clearance in the bite (**Fig. 9**).

Glycerin was then applied lightly to the area; Luxatemp (DMG America, Englewood, NJ) was injected into the initial mold of the patient's teeth, seated in the mouth for 2 minutes, and gently pulled out. Any excess material was cleaned from the area. The material was allowed a full 4 minutes to set, then removed and shaped outside the mouth (**Fig. 10**). Care was taken not to put pressure on the pontic site. The mesial aspect of teeth 7 and 9 was sounded to find the crest

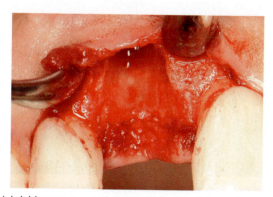

Fig. 7. Severe facial dehiscence approximating the apex of the socket.

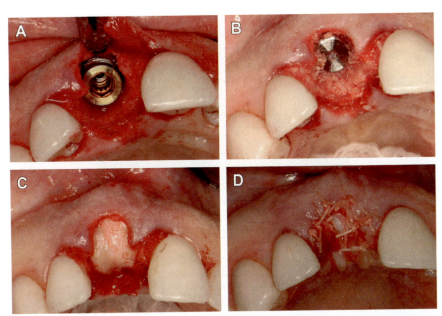

Fig. 8. (*A–D*) An immediate implant (NanoTite, 5 × 13 mm; BIOMET 3i, Palm Beach Gardens, FL) was stabilized in the residual socket and DFDBA was used to fill the gap and augment the facial dehiscence. A thick subepithelial connective tissue graft was used instead of a membrane to augment the soft tissue, improve primary closure, and attempt vertical augmentation to decrease the gingival discrepancy that existed.

of bone. Contact points were created roughly 4.5 to 5.0 mm long to ensure papillary regeneration. The bridge was then polished and cemented with TempBond Clear (Kerr Corporation, Orange, CA); excess cement was removed, and the bite was checked (**Fig. 11**).

At 10 weeks after implant surgery, facial soft tissue collapse was beginning to appear. A decision was made to perform a second thick subepithelial connective graft to get additional facial and vertical augmentation (**Fig. 12**).

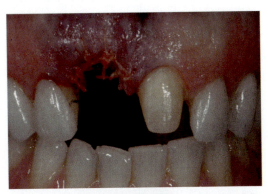

Fig. 9. Preparation was converted to a porcelain jacket, removing 1.5 mm circumferential and 1.5 mm incisally. The lingual was scooped out to provide adequate prosthetic clearance.

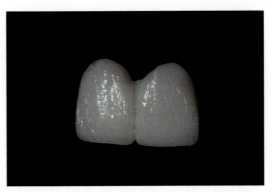

Fig. 10. Luxatemp was injected into the initial mold of the patient's teeth, seated in the mouth for 2 minutes, and gently pulled out.

A broad palatal to facial flap was performed using vertical incisions the distals of 7 and 9. Granulation tissue was noted over the dehiscence site, and a subepithelial connective tissue graft (SECTG) measuring 15 mm × 11 mm × 4 mm thick was recovered from the palate and stabilized over the implant. Primary closure was then achieved (**Figs. 13–15**).[4]

The provisional was adjusted by the restorative dentist to create light pressure and start sculpting an ovate pontic (**Figs. 16** and **17**).

Four weeks after the second SECTG, aesthetic crown lengthening was performed.

Aesthetic crown lengthening

Facial aesthetic design (FAD) was used to diagnose the proper clinical crown length. A maxillary cant existed with more gingival display present on the patient's right side than on her left. Teeth 3 to 14 were measured exactly, including initial tooth length, final tooth length, and any change to incisal edge position. The restorative dentist performed a live mock-up at the time of surgery to communicate visually to the periodontist the cant and gingival apices. Initial incisions were performed with a 15C blade to the final clinical crown length for each tooth, while preserving the interproximal tissue and avoiding the palatal tissue (**Fig. 18**).[5–8]

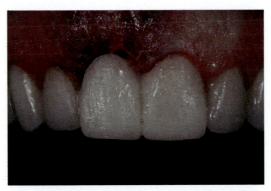

Fig. 11. The bridge was polished and cemented with TempBond Clear; excess cement was removed; and the bite was checked.

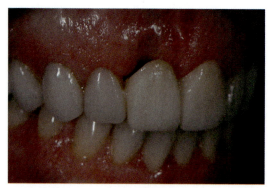

Fig. 12. Ten weeks after implant surgery, facial soft tissue collapse was beginning to appear.

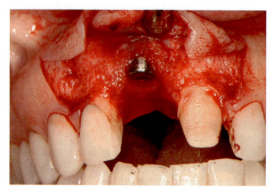

Fig. 13. Granulation tissue was noted over the dehiscence site.

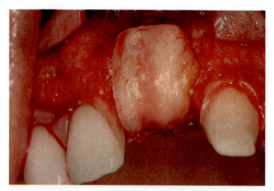

Fig. 14. An SECTG measuring 15 mm × 11 mm × 4 mm thick was recovered from the palate and stabilized over the implant.

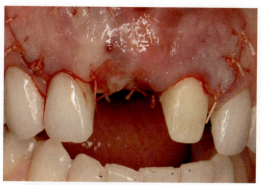

Fig. 15. Primary closure of the wound.

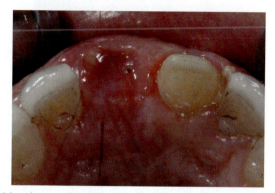

Fig. 16. The provisional was adjusted by the restorative dentist to create light pressure.

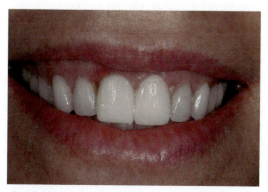

Fig. 17. The restorative dentist started sculpting an ovate pontic.

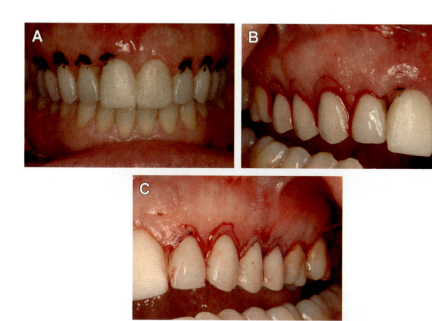

Fig. 18. (A–C) The patient had a maxillary cant, with more gingival display present on her right side than on her left side. Teeth numbers 3 to 14 were measured exactly, including initial tooth length, final tooth length, and any change to incisal edge position. Initial incisions were performed with a 15C blade to the final clinical crown length for each tooth, while preserving the interproximal tissue and avoiding the palatal tissue.

Full-thickness facial flaps were reflected for full osseous access. Both osteoplasty and ostectomy were performed for osseous correction (**Fig. 19**). In this patient, buttressing bone was present in the buccal corridors, which required osteoplasty to achieve the proper horizontal bone profile. Ostectomy was performed to give the proper vertical height and to prevent biologic width impingement. Enamel matrix derivative (Emdogain, Straumann USA LLC, Andover, MA) was applied to the root surfaces before closure to enhance gingival margin stability and wound healing. Primary closure was performed with advanced polyglactin 910 sutures (Vicryl Rapide, Ethicon, Inc, Somerville, NJ) using a figure 8 technique to place the gingival margin at its original position and keep it 3 mm from the osseous crest (**Fig. 20**).

RESTORATIVE PHASE OF TREATMENT
Preparation

At 8 weeks after surgery the patient returned to the restorative dentist to begin the restorative phase of treatment (**Fig. 21**). FAD principles were used to visualize the proper position of the smile.[9] A direct addition/reduction mock-up was done directly over the existing restorations in order to gain the final tooth position (**Fig. 22**). An alginate impression of this was taken and used as a stent in making the provisional.

Three carpules of Septocaine were administered from the second premolar to the second premolar. Preparations were then started directly through the addition/

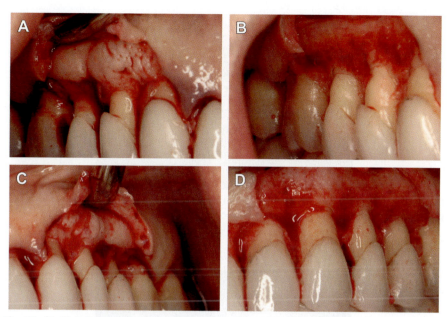

Fig. 19. (*A–D*) Full-thickness facial flaps were reflected for full osseous access. Both osteoplasty and ostectomy were performed for osseous correction.

reduction mock-up that was previously performed. Once ideal veneer preparations on teeth 4 to 7 and 11 to 13, as well as an all-ceramic crown preparation, were complete, the remaining ceramic from previous veneers was removed and the margins were finished (**Fig. 23**).

The implant was then uncovered using a diode laser. Care was taken not to cause lateral necrosis as a result of the laser being in contact with the tissue for too long (**Fig. 24**).[10] A PreFormance temporary abutment (BIOMET 3i) was then screwed in place and prepared for a crown at the level of the soft tissue (**Fig. 25**).

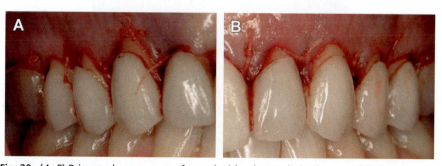

Fig. 20. (*A, B*) Primary closure was performed with advanced Vicryl sutures (Rapide), using a **figure 8** technique to place the gingival margin at its original position and keep it 3 mm from the osseous crest.

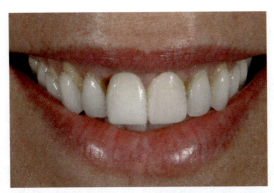

Fig. 21. At 8 weeks after surgery, the patient returned to the restorative dentist to begin provisionalization and the restorative phase of treatment.

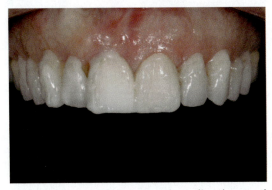

Fig. 22. A direct addition/reduction mock-up was done directly over the existing restorations in order to gain final tooth position.

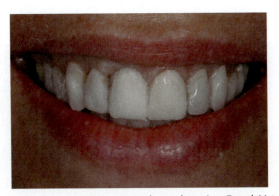

Fig. 23. Once ideal veneer preparations on teeth numbers 4 to 7 and 11 to 13 as well as an all-ceramic crown preparation were complete, the remaining ceramic from previous veneers was removed and margins were finished.

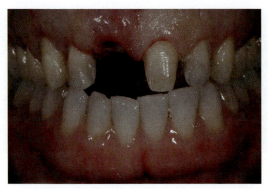

Fig. 24. The implant was then uncovered using a diode laser, being careful not to cause lateral necrosis from the laser being in contact with the tissue for too long.

Provisionalization

Provisionals were then fabricated using bis-acryl (Luxatemp) injected directly into an alginate impression of the addition/reduction mock-up. Glycerin was applied to the teeth, the alginate was seated, and the material was allowed to partially set for 2 minutes. The provisionals were pulled from the mouth and checked for adequate room of restorative material. Once adequate reduction was verified, the final impression was taken.[11]

Final Impression/Records/Temporization

Expasyl (Kerr Corporation) was placed into the sulcus and the provisionals were reseated to achieve both tissue retraction and hemostasis. This was left for 5 minutes. The provisional was removed, and the Expasyl was rinsed out completely with copious amounts of water. An impression coping was then screwed in to the 8 site. The teeth were dried, and a light body Impregum (3M, St. Paul, MN) was carefully syringed around the margins. For prevention of air bubbles, the tip of the syringe was not lifted out of the light-bodied impression material. Simultaneously, heavy body was

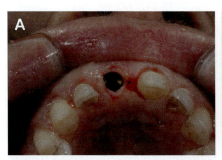
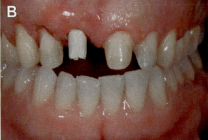

Fig. 25. (*A*, *B*) A PreFormance temporary abutment was then screwed in place and prepared for a crown at the level of the tissue.

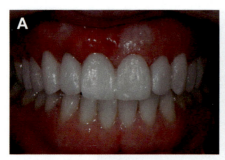
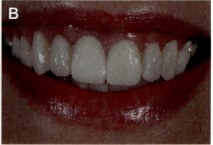

Fig. 26. (*A, B*) Photographic series of provisionals.

dispensed into a fitted tray and seated into the mouth. This was allowed to set for the recommended full 5 minutes before being removed.

An MIP bite was taken with Regisil (Dentsply, York, PA). Photographs of preparations as well as stump shades were taken. Temporaries were spot etched, bonded into place,[12] shaped, and finished in the mouth. The occlusion was adjusted as required. Photographs of the provisionals were taken (**Fig. 26**)[13] as well as measurements of central incisors. Shade selection was discussed with the patient. The records and a detailed lab script were sent to the dental technician.

Insertion

The patient returned in 1 week for insertion. Three carpules of Septocaine were administered. The temporaries were removed as well as the PreFormance abutment. The custom abutment was inserted; seating was confirmed by x-ray and torqued to 20 n/cm. All units, 4-13, were tried in with water (**Fig. 27**). Veneers and crowns were then prepared with silane and unfilled resin. The teeth were isolated with an OptraGate (Ivoclar Vivadent, Schaan, Lichtenstsein) and a total etch technique was used.[14] All veneers were inserted with B1 LuxaFlow light cure (DMG America, Englewood, NJ) as the luting cement, and both the implant crown and the all-ceramic crown on 9 were inserted with NX3 White Dual (Kerr Corporation). The restorations were cured, cleaned, and polished and the occlusion was checked (**Fig. 28**).

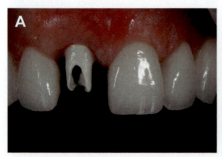
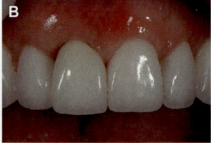

Fig. 27. (*A, B*) All units were tried in with water from numbers 4 to 13.

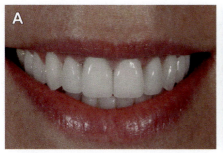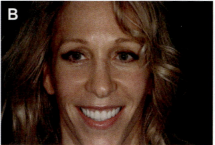

Fig. 28. (*A*, *B*) Restorations were bonded, cleaned, polished, and the occlusion was checked.

SUMMARY

This article reviews the traditional approach to the treatment of a complex interdisciplinary case and the importance of communication to achieve the ultimate perio-restorative interface. FAD was used to aid in the development of an aesthetic blueprint, so that soft and hard tissue discrepancies could be eliminated to improve the restorative aesthetic outcome and minimize the patient's facial asymmetry. In this patient, both hard and soft tissue regeneration and resection were required to achieve the required restorative parameters. Multiple surgical procedures were required to compensate for compromised gingival and bone levels for the single implant being placed in the position of tooth 8. A single surgical approach was used for the aesthetic crown lengthening. The elimination of excessive gingival display, gingival margin discrepancies, and the diagnosis and correction of the patient's maxillary cant are all derived from the aesthetic blueprint and the restorative and surgical parameters of FAD. The team approach is essential in achieving ideal aesthetics for an interdisciplinary treatment plan; when communication occurs properly, the aesthetic surgery can be considered a surgical component of the restorative therapy. Future articles should look at developing innovative strategies to streamline the treatment sequence.

REFERENCES

1. Ferrario VF, Poggio CE, Sforza C, et al. Distance from symmetry: a three-dimensional evaluation of facial asymmetry. J Oral Maxillofac Surg 1994;52: 1126–32.
2. Lazzara RJ. Immediate implant placement into extraction sites: surgical and restorative advantages. Int J Periodontics Restorative Dent 1989;9(5):332–43.
3. Gelb DA. Immediate implant surgery: three-year retrospective evaluation of 50 consecutive cases. Int J Oral Maxillofac Implants 1993;8(4):388–99.
4. Langer B, Langer L. Subepithelial connective tissue graft technique for root coverage. J Periodontol 1985;56(12):715–20.
5. Allen EP. Surgical crown lengthening for function and esthetics. Dent Clin North Am 1993;37:163–79.
6. Becker W, Ochsenbein C, Becker BE. Crown lengthening: the periodontal-restorative connection. Compend Contin Educ Dent 1998;19:239–40, 242, 244–46.
7. Lee EA. Aesthetic crown lengthening: classification, biologic rationale, and treatment planning considerations. Pract Proced Aesthet Dent 2004;16(10):769–78.
8. Garber DA, Salama MA. The aesthetic smile: diagnosis and treatment. Periodontol 2000 1996;11:18–28.

9. Calamia JR, Ciseros G, Levine JB, et al. Smile design and treatment planning with the help of a comprehensive esthetic evaluation form. Dent Clin North Am 2011; 55:187–209.

10. Lee EA. Laser-assisted crown lengthening procedures in the esthetic zone: contemporary guidelines and techniques. Contemporary Esthet 2006;10:42–9.

11. Gurel G. Predictable and precise tooth preparation techniques for PLVs in complex cases. Oral Health 2007;15–26.

12. McLaren EA. Porcelain veneer preparations: to prep or not to prep. Inside Dent 2006;2(4):76–9.

13. Radz G. Minimum thickness anterior porcelain restorations. Dent Clin North Am 2011;55:353–70.

14. Derand T, Treodson M. Effect of margin design, cement polymerization, and angle of loading stress in porcelain veneers. J Prosthet Dent 1999;82:518–24.

Restoration of the Anterior Segment in a Cleft Palate in Conjunction with Surgically Facilitated Orthodontic Therapy

CrossMark

An Interdisciplinary Approach

Chiann Fan Gibson, DMD[a,b,*], George A. Mandelaris, DDS, MS[c,d,e]

KEYWORDS

- Surgically facilitated orthodontic therapy (SFOT) • Restorative and cosmetic dentistry
- Cleft palate • Interdisciplinary

KEY POINTS

- Surgically facilitated orthodontic therapy can be an integral part of a comprehensive, interdisciplinary dentofacial therapy treatment plan that simultaneously addresses periodontal conditions, cosmetic/esthetic restorative space appropriation dilemmas, occlusion, and possibly airway-related improvements.
- Clear, consistent, and ongoing communication among restorative/cosmetic dentists, surgical specialists (dental and medical), patient, and family is essential to achieve optimal treatment outcomes.

CASE PRESENTATION

Patient Background

A healthy 26-year-old white woman presented to the restorative practice for esthetic improvement to her smile. She had resin-bonded veneers on teeth numbers 5, 6, 7, 8, and 12 and a resin-bonded Maryland bridge between numbers 9 and 11, spanning a unilateral alveolar oronasal fistula that was a sequel of unsuccessful unilateral cleft

Disclosure: The authors have no conflicts of interest.
[a] Private Practice, Restorative Dentistry, Naperville, IL, USA; [b] Department of Prosthodontics, Tufts School of Dental Medicine, Boston, MA, USA; [c] Private Practice, Periodontics and Dental Implant Surgery (Periodontal Medicine & Surgical Specialists, Ltd), Park Ridge, IL, USA; [d] Private Practice, Periodontics and Dental Implant Surgery (Periodontal Medicine & Surgical Specialists, Ltd), 1 South 224 Summit Avenue, Suite 205, Oakbrook Terrace, IL 60181, USA; [e] Department of Graduate Periodontics, University of Illinois College of Dentistry, Chicago, IL, USA
* Corresponding author. Smiles by Dr. Gibson, Promenade Dental of Naperville Illinois, 55 South Main Street, Suite 290, Naperville, IL 60540.
E-mail addresses: DrChiann@aol.com; Drchianngibson@gmail.com

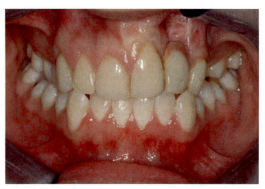

Fig. 1. Resin-bonded Maryland bridge 9 to 11 and resin-bonded veneers 6 to 8 (10 years old).

palate repair when she was 1 year old (**Figs. 1** and **2**). She was dissatisfied not only with the deteriorating esthetics of these restorations (which had been in place for approximately 10 years) and shifting of the bridge but also with her overall smile esthetics, and she desired improvement.

Medical history
The patient was in good systemic health.[1] Her medical history was unremarkable except for asthma, seasonal allergies, and a history of eczema. Her current medications included montelukast sodium, cetirizine, mometasone furoate monohydrate nasal spray, and eye drops (allergy related), which she took to manage her allergic/asthmatic symptoms.

Dental history
The patient was born with a left unilateral cleft lip and palate. Although the lip repair was successful at age 3 months, the attempted closure of the bony palatal cleft at age 1 year was not. The remaining bony and soft tissue defect extended through the alveolar process and oral mucosa, leaving an alveolar communication between the oral and nasal cavities (oronasal fistula) in the number 10 position.

The craniofacial defect created by the unilateral (left) maxillary cleft resulted in an hourglass-shaped upper arch form and a bilateral crossbite (**Figs. 3** and **4**). She

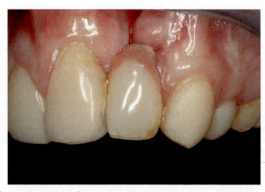

Fig. 2. Unsuccessful unilateral cleft palate repair. Failing resin-bonded Maryland bridge.

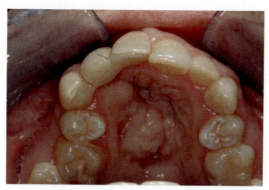

Fig. 3. Occlusal view of maxillary arch showing hourglass-shaped form.

was originally seen by the treating periodontist in 2004 for management of a recession defect, which was corrected by a connective tissue graft alone via a tunneling procedure.

Following connective tissue graft healing, her dentist at that time managed cosmetic concerns by composite bonding in the anterior maxilla.

Figs. 5–7 show the pretreatment appearance of the dentition at roughly 6 years after treatment, showing the resin-bonded bridge in place at the start of current treatment (see **Figs. 1–4**). **Fig. 8** shows a full-face pretreatment view of the patient; **Fig. 9** shows her initial full-mouth radiographic series from February 2010. The relapse in recession underscores the biological short-coming of connective tissue grafting for root coverage purposes, which results in a long-junctional epithelium compared with the more desirable outcome of periodontal regeneration (cementum, alveolar bone, and periodontal ligament).[2]

She had undergone 2 previous periods of orthodontic treatment, during which teeth numbers 4 and 13 were extracted, and numbers 1 and 16 were retained (numbers 17 and 32 are retained and impacted). The resulting occlusion comprised an Angle class II molar relationship on the right (**Fig. 10**), and a class I relationship on the left (in the area of the cleft-related arch deficit; **Fig. 11**). Her history also included alveolus repair, palate repair including velopharyngeal flap, rib grafting (as part of the attempted cleft repair), and alar and lip revisions; a noticeable alar discrepancy remains on the left side (see **Figs. 1, 3,** and **8**).

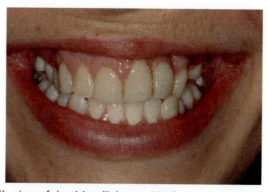

Fig. 4. Frontal smile view of dentition (February 2010).

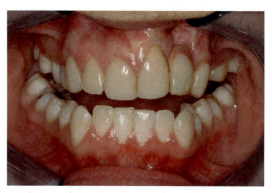

Fig. 5. Frontal retracted view of dentition (February 2010).

Overall, her oral hygiene was good, and she remains on a preventive recall schedule with adult prophylaxis and oral examination at 6-month intervals.

DIAGNOSTIC AIDS

The initial consultation for the interdisciplinary team described in this article took place in February 2010, involving the patient, restorative dentist, periodontist, and orthodontist; a standard full-mouth radiographic series and high-quality diagnostic casts were obtained.

Pretreatment cone beam computed tomography (CBCT) was also obtained as a part of diagnostics and treatment planning. In addition, secondary CBCT was secured for comparison with posttreatment results at 4 months after surgically facilitated orthodontic therapy (SFOT).

Fig. 12 shows a problem-management algorithm, with various dentoalveolar and orthodontic considerations that must be considered for SFOT treatment planning.

SMILE EVALUATION

After the initial group consultation, a pretreatment orthodontic setup was performed in the orthodontist's office in April 2010, consisting of panoramic and lateral cephalometric radiographs, plus a tracing and analysis (**Figs. 13–15**). This setup was followed

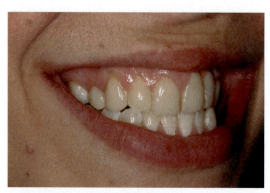

Fig. 6. Right smile; February 2010 (before surgery).

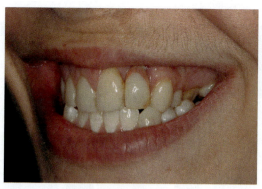

Fig. 7. Left smile; February 2010 (before surgery).

by a diagnostic wax-up, which was performed by the laboratory technologist (Smiles Inc, Boise, ID) working with the restorative dentist, to provide a preview of the smile design based on the results the patient desired.

Diagnosis and Treatment History

The restorative dentist had first seen the patient in February 2010 for the initial consult; the following month her father accompanied her for a follow-up visit. The outcome of that visit's discussion then encompassed the collaborative involvement of a periodontist and an orthodontist for an integrated treatment planning approach (see **Fig. 12**).

After orthodontic bracketing and arch wires were placed (with the initial intention of erupting number 9 and ultimately extracting it, leading to placement of an implant with a cantilevered pontic into number 10 position), a discussion took place regarding changing the treatment plan, which resulted in modification of the initial diagnostic wax-up.

The scenario expressed here underscores the interdisciplinary team approach of constant evaluation and reevaluation analysis that is performed during treatment of such cases to ensure that the outcome goal meets or exceeds the best possible biological, functional, and esthetic goals for the patient.

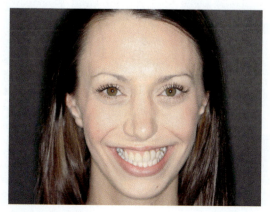

Fig. 8. Full-face pretreatment view.

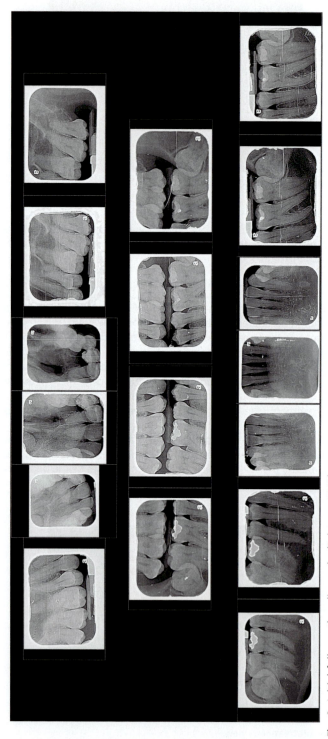

Fig. 9. Initial full-mouth radiographs (February 2010).

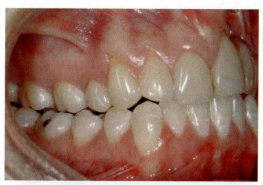

Fig. 10. Occlusion, right side, showing class II molar relationship and crossbite.

Cone beam computed tomography imaging

CBCT imaging of the patient's maxillary arch was performed before initiating SFOT and as a part of diagnostics, then at 4 months after completion of SFOT, to validate and verify bone augmentation results as well as to compare the corticotomy-assisted tooth position after regional acceleratory phenomenon (RAP) (**Fig. 16**).

SEQUENCING OF TREATMENT (PHASES)
Treatment Sequence Overview

In February 2010, after conducting the initial patient consultation, comprehensive examination, charting, and prophylaxis, the cosmetic dentist referred the patient to a periodontist (whom she had seen several years earlier in connection with aesthetic correction of the soft tissue cleft defect). The periodontist in turn suggested that she see an orthodontist, who ultimately proposed the SFOT treatment sequence.

In March 2010, both the patient and her father returned for another consultation with the cosmetic dentist, to review the wax-up and discuss her aesthetic goals.

In June 2010, the cosmetic/restorative dentist arranged a joint consultation with the periodontist and orthodontist regarding formation of an interdisciplinary team.

An initial step in the treatment plan was endodontic treatment of tooth number 9 in July 2010, because of the amount of reduction anticipated in preparing this tooth for

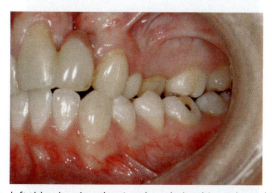

Fig. 11. Occlusion, left side, showing class I molar relationship and crossbite.

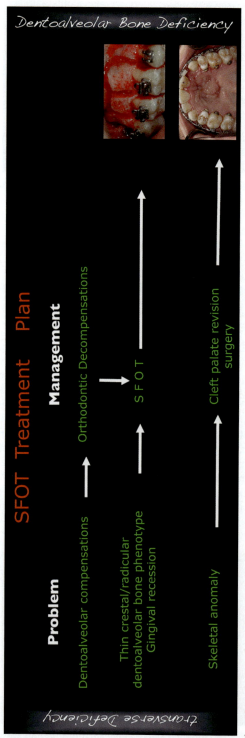

Fig. 12. Integrated treatment plan with periodontal-orthodontal collaboration using SFOT.

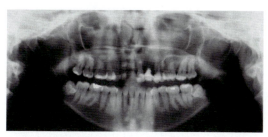

Fig. 13. Panoramic radiograph (2010, before treatment).

esthetic restorations. Orthodontic treatment was started in August 2010. During the orthodontic phase, the pontic in position number 10 was incorporated into the bracketing.

A 3-month to 4-month prophylaxis schedule was instituted in April 2011 because of plaque accumulation and to reduce inflammation in the presence of tooth movement, with emphasis on self-performed oral hygiene recommendations. The next prophylaxis was done in September 2011 (at which point the cosmetic dentist obtained photographs to update the periodontist on the patient's orthodontic progress) followed by another cleaning in December 2011, when she expressed a desire to have the orthodontic bracketing removed at this time. By her recare appointment in June 2012, the SFOT surgical phase and bone grafting of the posterior maxillary segments had been completed. The cosmetic dentist obtained new photographs, which were sent to the orthodontist and periodontist. **Figs. 17–19** show the 4-month post-SFOT arch form changes and periodontal phenotype transformation.

At this stage, there was discussion of connective tissue (CT) graft in position number 9, and the decision was weighed as to retaining this endodontically treated tooth as an alternative to extraction.

Another group consultation meeting took place in July 2012 for restorative treatment planning; the possibility of cantilevering the pontic in position number 10 from number 11 was discussed, because of the questionable prognosis of tooth number 9 and the possibility of moving to an implant. Based on evaluation and discussion during this

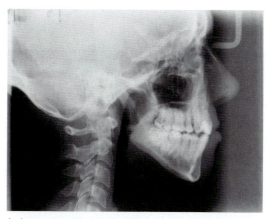

Fig. 14. Lateral cephalometric radiograph. Orthodontic work-up.

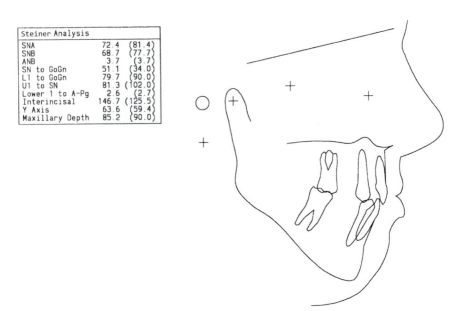

Steiner Analysis		
SNA	72.4	(81.4)
SNB	68.7	(77.7)
ANB	3.7	(3.7)
SN to GoGn	51.1	(34.0)
L1 to GoGn	79.7	(90.0)
U1 to SN	81.3	(102.0)
Lower 1 to A-Pg	2.6	(2.7)
Interincisal	146.7	(125.5)
Y Axis	63.6	(59.4)
Maxillary Depth	85.2	(90.0)

Fig. 15. Cephalometric tracing (Steiner analysis). Orthodontic work-up.

group consult, the option of placing a bridge from number 9 to number 11 became the final restorative goal because the periodontal prognosis associated with number 9 was determined to be fair.

A new photographic series was taken in August 2012 to better visualize and assess the number 10 position pontic site. Then, a cosmetic wax-up was done based on the final decision to retain number 9 for a bridge spanning numbers 9 to 11 (August 2012). Whitening trays were also fabricated in August 2012 in conjunction with an in-office whitening procedure (Venus, Heraeus Kulzer GmbH, South Bend, IN). The patient continued to use at-home trays for the lower arch to continue whitening until her final impressions were obtained.

By September 2012 the patient had reviewed all treatment objectives; approved the cosmetic wax-up; signed the consent for cosmetic restorations and goals; and, after

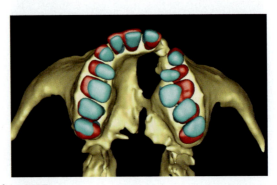

Fig. 16. CBCT before SFOT.

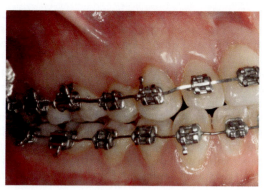

Fig. 17. Right lateral view 4 months after SFOT.

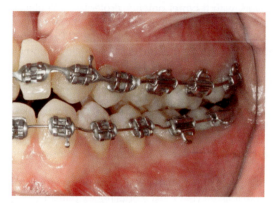

Fig. 18. Left lateral view 4 months after SFOT.

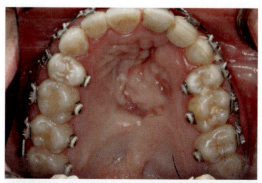

Fig. 19. Occlusal view 4 months after SFOT showing arch form changes and periodontal phenotype transformation.

pretreatment photographs were obtained and shared with the orthodontist and periodontist and an updated full-mouth radiographic series was obtained, the treatment team and patient moved forward with tooth preparation and provisionalization (which extended to February 2013, when the final restorations were placed).

Evaluation of occlusion and function as well as routine office visits were done between October and early December 2012, at which point new provisionals were constructed to accommodate site development of the number 10 pontic position (**Fig. 20**). The periodontist reevaluated the tissues in the left anterior segment postsurgically in January 2013 and observed normal healing of the graft. In consultation with the restorative doctor and while the patient was in provisionals, final crown lengthening was performed in conjunction with a rotated palatal pedicle epithelialized CT graft in an attempt to gain an improved vertical soft tissue mass and form at the number 10 site.[3]

In February 2013, final maxillary and mandibular full-arch polyvinyl siloxane impressions were obtained, together with a bite registration. Photographs and stump shade were obtained for laboratory use.

Overall, after the interdisciplinary treatment with SFOT, the interincisal angle was successfully improved, with a better anterior protected articulation scheme, and, in theory, a more patent airway because of the increased oral cavity volume and associated increased in oral cavity/tongue volume ratio.[4] SFOT provided a novel approach to treating a complex problem to afford a highly esthetic outcome.

Restorative/cosmetic dentistry

After completion of SFOT and team approval of the restorative treatment plan (which consisted of all-ceramic [e.max] restorations on teeth numbers 5, 6, 7, 9 to 11, and 12), a diagnostic wax-up was done for the periodontist to use and work backward to see how and what surgery would be required to meet the prosthetic outcome requirements/goals. The wax-up was done on diagnostic casts done after orthodontia.

Such a wax-up is a piece of the puzzle that many practitioners try to avoid; this can be a pitfall in that a preliminary view can be obtained of patient preferences that can be captured in provisionalization. Then, in the provisional phase, patients can become accustomed to the intricacies of the smile contour represented by the provisional, and make any modifications based on their individual preferences, which may shift over the course of time during treatment. The cosmetic wax-up was reviewed and accepted by the patient.

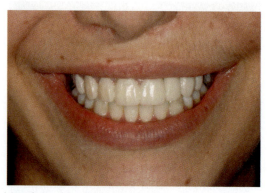

Fig. 20. Final provisionals in place (December 2012).

The restorative treatment plan comprised several phases, including provisionalization. Provisionalization provides the clinician the opportunity to query the patient on specifics of smile design and elicit feedback that can be used to design the final restoration, which is a different material and reflects/transmits light differently from the provisional (see **Figs. 20** and **21**).

Because the patient also reported a history of nocturnal bruxism, she was given a maxillary hard exterior/soft interior occlusal guard (comfort guard) to wear at night to protect her dentition and newly placed restorations.

Laboratory specifications

After casts were created from impressions, and the diagnostic wax-up was performed to idealize shape, position, and form with function; all-ceramic crowns were fabricated for teeth numbers 5, 6, 7, 8, and 12; tooth number 9, number 10 pontic, and number 11 comprised an all-ceramic bridge. Custom characterizations were done using Empress universal shade 110/120 and e.max Ceram Glaze Paste to produce appropriate gloss in white and pink ceramics. Because of proclination of tooth number 7, adjustments were made to harmonize as much as possible with mandibular occlusion and incorporate American Academy of Cosmetic Dentistry (AACD) smile design principles.

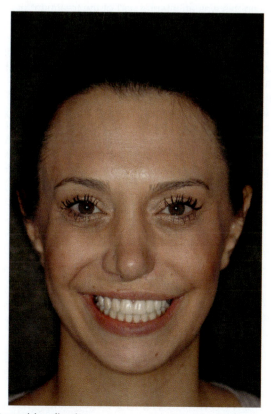

Fig. 21. Headshot provisionalization.

Pink tissue porcelain was used to blend with the color of the natural dentition. e.max Ceram IG3 powders were used as the base layer for intensity, e.max Ceram G3 was then layered over the base layer, and e.max glaze paste was used for finish to a gloss.

Smile design principles

The restorative/cosmetic dentist analyzed the patient's smile according to smile design parameters established in connection with the AACD accreditation criteria,[5] and as discussed/interpreted in a recent review by Mistry.[6] In addition, The AACD guide to accreditation criteria, *Contemporary Concepts in Smile Design: Diagnosis and Treatment Evaluation in Comprehensive Cosmetic Dentistry* discusses how the smile line, in conjunction with other factors, helps determine the incisal edge position, influences the lengths of the maxillary central incisors, and identifies an ideal or pleasing range of 10 to 12 mm for length of maxillary centrals.

In this patient's case, the parameters assessed included axial line angles and elements of the Golden Proportion, notably the avoidance of square-looking teeth, as well as ensuring that the interpupillary eye line is parallel with the plane of occlusion. This principle also focuses on symmetry of central incisors proceeding distally, in which the usual ratio is 10-mm length and 8-mm width, with broadening discrepancies progressing distally.

Considerable negative space was present in the buccal corridors. Because the basic goal of cosmetic dentistry is to impart fullness to the arch form along the buccal corridors, addressing this was an integral part of the treatment plan.

Gingival esthetics

This patient's initial gingival height reflected excessive gingival display (EGD; the so-called gummy smile), in addition to the pronounced recession defect on the facial aspect of tooth number 9 (see **Figs. 4**, **7**, **8**; **Figs. 22** and **23**).

After reevaluation of the cosmetic wax-up, the team discussed with the patient various options for correction of her EGD; lip repositioning surgery would not have been an option for this patient case because of the vestibular/alveolar defects resulting from the cleft, and thus a predictable result was unlikely. Hence, she decided on the option of esthetic clinical crown lengthening on teeth numbers 5 to 12, which the periodontist performed in November 2012 at the same time as the rotated palatal pedicle epithelialized CT graft.

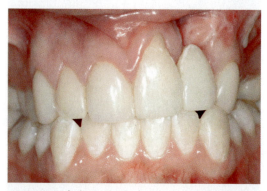

Fig. 22. Pretreatment, retracted view, gingival esthetics, showing severe recession defect, facial aspect of tooth no. 9.

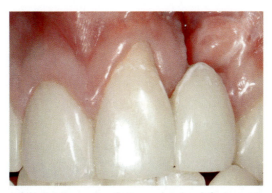

Fig. 23. Recession defect, tooth no. 9, soft tissue alveolar defect, position no. 10.

The original treatment plan included erupting tooth number 9, treating it endodontically, and placing an implant in this position with a cantilevered lateral incisor.

Although placing an implant was ultimately rejected, endodontic treatment was required at the outset to enable the eruption of tooth number 9 because of the required reduction to create vertical space in order for eruption to occur, and the team wished to avoid pulpal problems during orthodontia, which might have jeopardized the facial bone. Therefore, endodontic treatment was completed before starting orthodontia (**Fig. 24**).

Tooth number 9 and the bone surrounding it were determined to be sound, and thus suitable for use as an abutment for the bridge from numbers 9 to 11, hence the team decision was made in July 2012 to retain tooth number 9. Its prognosis was determined as fair to good in the short and long terms.[7]

The treatment plan required approximately 3 years, including the period of SFOT and alveolar cleft repair, before cementation of final bridge.

Fig. 25 shows the initial cosmetic result in the first year. **Figs. 26–31** show the final esthetic views 3 years after initiation of the interdisciplinary treatment plan (June 2013). **Fig. 32** shows the 3-year full-mouth radiographic series.

DISCUSSION

The overall objective of the interdisciplinary approach used in this case had the focal point of completing SFOT in order to achieve the foundation that the interdisciplinary treatment team needed to provide the final result desired by the patient.[8] The interdisciplinary approach has received considerable recent attention in the literature, notably with regard to its importance in interactions between restorative dentists, orthodontists, and periodontists,[9] minimizing the occurrence of quality-of-life issues in patients with cleft palates,[10] and providing a more idealized treatment scenario even in the context of a nonsurgical approach to cleft management.[11]

By integrating SFOT with such an interdisciplinary approach, we were able to provide this patient with an outcome that has historically only been achieved with orthognathic surgery. SFOT increases oral cavity volume, produces better anterior tongue posturing opportunities, gains space to facilitate optimal esthetic and restorative dentistry, and achieves occlusion goals that help to maintain postorthodontic stability.[12–21] In addition, SFOT allows the orthodontic walls to be redefined and effectively changes the periodontal phenotype of at-risk periodontiums and allows patients the benefit of a reduction in orthodontic treatment time.[22–24]

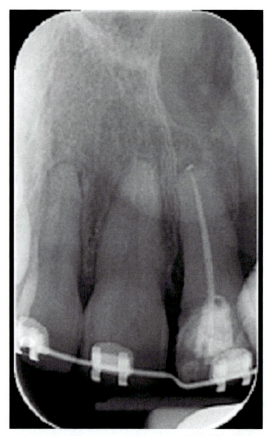

Fig. 24. Periapical radiograph of root canal treatment final fill, tooth no. 9.

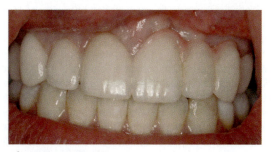

Fig. 25. Final view of anterior segment.

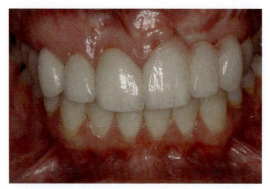

Fig. 26. Final esthetics, frontal retracted view, maximum intercuspation.

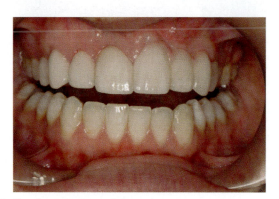

Fig. 27. Final esthetics, frontal retracted view, open.

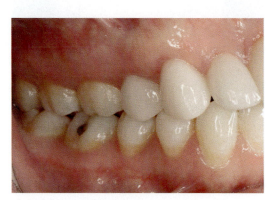

Fig. 28. Right lateral view 3 years after surgery.

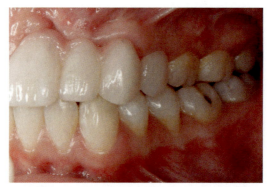

Fig. 29. Left lateral view 3 years after surgery.

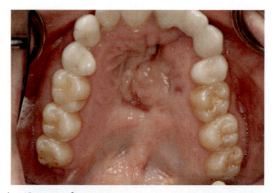

Fig. 30. Occlusal view 3 years after surgery.

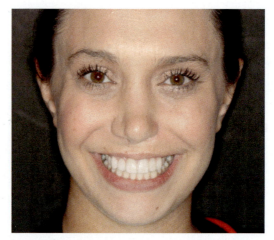

Fig. 31. Headshot 3 years after surgery.

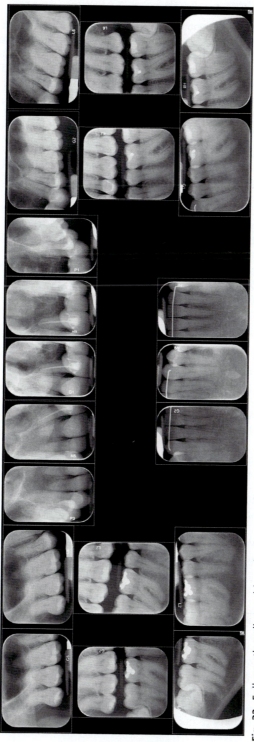

Fig. 32. Full-mouth radiographic series 3 years after surgery.

ACKNOWLEDGMENTS

The authors thank the patient for participating in the coordinated interdisciplinary treatment; Dave Morris, MD, plastic and reconstructive surgeon at the University of Illinois Medical Center, Chicago, IL, for performing the cleft palate repair; and Scott A. Saunders, DDS, ELS, CMPP at DMWE Dental and Medical Writing and Editing, LLC, Royersford, PA, for professional dental and medical writing services in the preparation of the article.

REFERENCES

1. ASA Physical Status Classification System. Available at: https://http://www.asahq.org/clinical/physicalstatus.htm.
2. McGuire MK, Scheyer ET, Schupach P. Growth factor-mediated treatment of recession defects: a randomized controlled trial and histologic and microcomputed tomography examination. J Periodontol 2009;80(4):550.
3. Stimmelmayr M, Allen EP, Gernet W, et al. Treatment of gingival recession in the anterior mandible using tunnel technique and a combination of epithelialized-subepithelial connective tissue graft- a case series. Int J Periodontics Restorative Dent 2011;31(2):165–73.
4. Iida-Kondo C, Yoshino N, Kurabayashi T, et al. Comparison of tongue volume/oral cavity volume ration between obstructive sleep apnea syndrome patients and normal adults using magnetic resonance imaging. J Med Dent Sci 2006;53:119–26.
5. Dentistry AAoC. Contemporary concepts in smile design: global esthetics. Journal of Cosmetic Dentistry 2014;29(4):132–4.
6. Mistry S. Principles of smile design-demystified. Journal of Cosmetic Dentistry 2012;28(2):116–24.
7. McGuire MK, Nunn ME. Prognosis versus actual outcome. II. The effectiveness of clinical parameters in developing an accurate prognosis. J Periodontol 1996;67(7):658–65.
8. Roblee RD, Bolding SL, Landers JM. Surgically facilitated orthodontic therapy: a new tool for optimal interdisciplinary results. Compend Contin Educ Dent 2009;30(5):264–75.
9. Gottesman E. Periodontal-restorative collaboration: the basis for interdisciplinary success in partially edentulous patients. Compend Contin Educ Dent 2012;33(7):478–82.
10. Guerrero CA. Cleft lip and palate surgery: 30 years follow-up. Ann Maxillofac Surg 2012;2(2):153–7.
11. Ma QL, Conley RS, Wu T, et al. Interdisciplinary treatment for an adult with a unilateral cleft lip and palate. Am J Orthod Dentofacial Orthop 2014;146(2):238–48.
12. Kole H. Surgical operations on the alveolar ridge to correct occlusal abnormalities. Oral Surg Oral Med Oral Pathol 1959;12(5):515–529 concl.
13. Frost HM. The biology of fracture healing. An overview for clinicians. Part I. Clin Orthop Relat Res 1989;(248):283–93.
14. Frost HM. The biology of fracture healing. An overview for clinicians. Part II. Clin Orthop Relat Res 1989;(248):294–309.
15. Wilcko WM, Wilcko T, Bouquot JE, et al. Rapid orthodontics with alveolar reshaping: two case reports of decrowding. Int J Periodontics Restorative Dent 2001;21(1):9–19.

16. Wilcko MT, Wilcko WM, Marquez MG, et al. The contribution of periodontics to or-thodontic therapy. In: Dibart S, editor. Practical advanced periodontal surgery. edition. Copenhagen (Denmark): Blackwell Munksgaard; 2007. p. 23–50.
17. Hoogeveen EJ, Jansma J, Ren Y. Surgically facilitated orthodontic treatment: a systematic review. Am J Orthod Dentofacial Orthop 2014;145(4 Suppl):S51–64.
18. Wilcko MT, Wilcko WM, Pulver JJ, et al. Accelerated osteogenic orthodontics technique: a 1-stage surgically facilitated rapid orthodontic technique with alve-olar augmentation. J Oral Maxillofac Surg 2009;67(10):2149–59.
19. Shoreibah EA, Ibrahim SA, Attia MS, et al. Clinical and radiographic evaluation of bone grafting in corticotomy-facilitated orthodontics in adults. J Int Acad Periodontol 2012;14(4):105–13.
20. Shoreibah EA, Salama AE, Attia MS, et al. Corticotomy-facilitated orthodontics in adults using a further modified technique. J Int Acad Periodontol 2012;14(4): 97–104.
21. Makki L, Ferguson DJ, Wilcko MT, et al. Mandibular irregularity index stability following alveolar corticotomy and grafting: a 10-year preliminary study: Mandibular Irregularity Index Stability. Angle Orthod 2014. [Epub ahead of print].
22. Gauthier C, Voyer R, Paquette M, et al. Periodontal effects of surgically assisted rapid palatal expansion evaluated clinically and with cone-beam computerized tomography: 6-month preliminary results. Am J Orthod Dentofacial Orthop 2011;139(4 Suppl):S117–28.
23. Handelman CS. The anterior alveolus: its importance in limiting orthodontic treat-ment and its influence on the occurrence of iatrogenic sequelae. Angle Orthod 1996;66(2):95–109 [discussion: 109–10].
24. Kapila S, Conley RS, Harrell WE Jr. The current status of cone beam computed tomography imaging in orthodontics. Dentomaxillofac Radiol 2011;40(1):24–34.

Index

Note: Page numbers of article titles are in **boldface** type.